GEOI D0441735

August 1, 2001

Dear Nancy,

Barbara and I have always admired your courage and determination, but we really did not appreciate everything you have accomplished until we read "Winning the Race."

This book is a wonderful testament to the love you had for your sister, and to your tenacity when faced with your own cancer challenge. If all of us faced adversity with your kind of "can do" attitude, then this would be a very different world.

Most importantly, this book will help save lives. You have given women a "how to" on dealing with breast cancer. It's a wonderful gift to all of us.

We've always been proud of you for everything you accomplished through The Susan G. Komen Breast Cancer Foundation. The book just adds to the incredible legacy you have built for your sister – and for you. Thanks for all your hard work in the cancer field, and we look forward to working with you in the future. With dedicated people such as yourself on the cancer team, I know that one day we'll beat this horrible disease.

With all best wishes,

G Bush

Nancy Brinker
The Susan G. Komen Breast Cancer Foundation
5005 LBJ Freeway
Suite 250
Dallas, Texas 75244

P. O. BOX 79798 · HOUSTON, TEXAS 77279-9798

ENDORSEMENTS

"*Winning* is a testament to the courage and conviction of Nancy Brinker's battle against breast cancer and her determination to take it out of whispered conversations and into a public arena to be challenged and, hopefully, cured. Hers is a story that will inspire everyone ever touched by this horrible disease. We at Yoplait are honored to have worked with Nancy to make a healthy difference in people's lives."
Ian Friendly, President, Yoplait U.S.A.

"Nancy Brinker provides readers with a powerful new guide to dealing with breast cancer, and proves once again that knowledge and determination are the most powerful tools for overcoming adversity, a lesson everyone—personally affected by breast cancer or not—can learn from."
Jacques Nasser, President and CEO of Ford Motor Company

"Anyone who has met Nancy Brinker, read of her work, participated in activities of the Susan G. Komen Breast Cancer Foundation has already been nearly overwhelmed by her. But this book, which chronicles, informs, educates, inspires, goes beyond anything we knew before . . . a *brilliant* tome that will surely accomplish Nancy's wish . . . to empower women with breast cancer and their loved ones to understand and become total partners in the treatment of the disease."
Helen Gurley Brown, Editor Cosmopolitan International

"This book is invaluable to the health and well-being of every woman, young and old. I'd recommend it to my mother, sister, family members and friends as a must read. Susan and Nancy's stories are not only inspiring, they've enlightened the world about breast cancer and subsequently empowered us all."
Bobbi Brown, Global Beauty Authority and Leading Makeup Artist

"Nancy Brinker has done it again and shown us why she is such a great leader in the fight against breast cancer. *Winning the Race: Taking Charge of Breast Cancer* is a great resource, tool, and inspiration to help patients and their families beat breast cancer."
John D. Minna, M.D., Director, Hamon Center for Therapeutic Oncology Research at University of Texas Southwestern Medical Center, Dallas, TX.

"This book will make you weep. But it will also inspire you and inform you. Nancy Brinker has written movingly about her sister's fight with breast cancer, her own fight with this disease, and her recovery. I was completely engrossed, touched, and moved."
Barbara Taylor Bradford, Best-Selling Novelist

"*Winning The Race: Taking Charge of Breast Cancer*, should be in every home in the country. Nancy Brinker takes the mystery out of the diagnosis and treatment of breast cancer in easy to understand terms punctuated with real life examples. This is a must read for ALL women and or loved ones of women who are diagnosed with breast cancer."

Marilyn Tucker Quayle, Wife of Former Vice President Dan Quayle

"This beautifully written and well-researched book could only have come from the mind and heart of Nancy Brinker. She has fought the war against breast cancer like no other person I know, and this book is the powerful result of her hard won knowledge. Just like Nancy, I've had breast cancer, and just like Nancy, I've lost a sister much too early in life. Either event can shatter your life, or it can empower you to make every day count . . . and to make a difference. With this extraordinary book, Nancy Brinker continues to honor her beloved sister . . . and to make a very large difference in the world."

Peggy Fleming Jenkins, 1968 Olympic Gold Medalist/ABC Sports Commentator

"I wish *Winning the Race, Taking Charge of Breast Cancer*" had been available to my family when my sister was diagnosed with breast cancer. Nancy's insights and sensitivity about her personal journey would have been a valuable companion to all of us. Bravo, Nancy, for your honesty and hard work. This is a must for men and women in the fight to eradicate breast cancer."

Marvin Hamlisch, Composer

"Taking charge of breast cancer is exactly what Nancy Brinker and the Susan G. Komen Breast Cancer Foundation have done for the last 20 years. The next 20 years will bring a profound celebration to the charge. Then Nancy and the Foundation will be writing about breast cancer's cure . . . not just the cause!!!"

Ellen Rohde, President, V.F. Intimates Coalition, V.F. Corporation

"The Susan G. Komen Breast Cancer Foundation is a beacon of hope for breast cancer patients and their families. Visionary leadership mixed with collaboration between advocates, scientists, and clinicians has permanently changed the breast cancer landscape. The Komen Foundation's Race for the Cure celebrates the lives of cancer survivors while underwriting excellent research and supporting community-based breast health education and breast cancer screening and treatment projects for the medically underserved."

Tommy G. Thompson, Secretary of Health and Human Services

Winning the Race

TAKING CHARGE OF BREAST CANCER

My Personal Story and Every
Woman's Guide to Wellness

by

Nancy G. Brinker

with

Chriss Winston

All royalties will be paid to the Susan G. Komen Breast Cancer Foundation.

TAPESTRY PRESS
Irving, Texas

Tapestry Press
3649 Conflans Road
Suite 103
Irving, TX 75061

Printed in the United States of America

05 04 03 02 01   5 4 3 2 1

Library of Congress Cataloging-in-Publication Data
Brinker, Nancy.
   Winning the race : taking charge of breast cancer : my personal
story and every woman's guide to wellness / by Nancy G. Brinker with
Chriss Anne Winston.
      p. cm.
Includes bibliographical references and index.
   ISBN 1-930819-05-6
   1. Breast—Cancer—Popular works. 2. Susan G. Komen Breast
Cancer Foundation. 3. Brinker, Nancy—Health. I. Winston, Chriss
Anne, 1948-
II. Title.
RC280.B8 B734 2001
616.99'449—dc21
                                        2001004328

Book design and layout by
D. & F. Scott Publishing,Inc.
N. Richland Hills, Texas

Cover by D. & F. Scott Publishing, Inc.
and Gavos and Helms Design

Associate Editor: Sloane Burke-Baty

CONTENTS

DEDICATION

To my sister, Suzy. The years have not broken our bond nor dimmed our promise. I still miss her every day of my life.

To my wonderful son, Eric, and my loving parents, Ellie and Marvin Goodman, who have always been the "wind beneath my wings."

To Suzy's own—Stephanie, Scott, and Maddie. She would be so proud.

And to the millions of Komen "angels" who have walked and run; cried and laughed; who broke the silence and made a difference in the lives of so many others.

Foreword

More than twenty-five years ago now, I was diagnosed with breast cancer. Like any woman facing this terrible disease, I was devastated. So was my family. But at the time, we weren't just any family. In September 1974, my address was 1600 Pennsylvania Avenue; so when I got the news that I would need a mastectomy, I had to make an important decision both as a woman and as first lady. Should I deal with this most personal illness in a private way, or share the news of my breast cancer with the American people? Back then you just didn't talk about breast cancer in "polite company." It was a much different era, and it was a difficult decision for me as it is for every woman. After much soul searching, my family and I decided to tell the world that I had breast cancer. Little did I realize that as first lady I

> "We must accept finite disappointment, but never lose infinite hope."
> Dr. Martin Luther King, Jr.

had a unique ability to focus attention on a disease that was killing tens of thousands of women every year and striking hundreds of thousands more. As a result, I felt I had a responsibility to use my personal situation, difficult though it was, as an opportunity to educate people about the need for more research and the importance of early detection.

Going public was not easy, but I learned a lot about myself: what I could handle and how much so many caring people had to give. I also learned that hope and humor are two "medicines" you literally can't live without. My family was always there for me, cheering me on, keeping me upbeat and smiling, but I found they needed my strength, too.

A couple of days after my surgery, I was taking a short walk down the hospital corridor when one of the Secret Service agents let me know that Jerry was on his way up. I ducked into my room and grabbed a "get-well" football I had received from the Washington Redskins signed by every member of the team. I got back to the hallway just in time to see the doors of the elevator open and my husband, the president, step out. "Catch!" I shouted and sent a wobbly pass his direction. He managed a respectable catch, but the awed expression on his face had the nurses and me in stitches. Of course, my husband and the doctor did not find my athletics funny, and the doctor promptly ordered me back to bed in no uncertain terms.

There were plenty of tears, too; but I realized early on that attitude is so important to recovery. My outcome was a happy one. A quarter of century later, I am grateful to be alive, but my joy is tempered with the knowledge that during this same time, more than a million women weren't as lucky as I was.

One of those was a woman named Suzy Goodman Komen, a beautiful young mother in Peoria, Illinois, who faced the same terrible news just three years after my diagnosis. For Suzy and her family—especially her younger sister, Nancy—breast cancer was the last thing they imagined would change their lives so dramatically. Despite a valiant effort, Suzy lost her battle. However, her fight and her last wish that no other woman should go through her ordeal inspired her sister, Nancy Brinker, to embark on what has been a twenty-year journey to eradicate breast cancer as a life-threatening disease.

Winning the Race: Taking Charge of Breast Cancer is their story and perhaps the prologue to yours as well. It is a testament to Nancy Brinker's love for her very special sister and to her strength and courage when faced with her own breast cancer diagnosis. Defeat is not in Nancy Brinker's vocabulary. She began her journey with nothing but an unshakeable determination to keep her promise to Suzy—a world without breast cancer. Through sheer will, Nancy created, in Suzy's memory, the Susan G. Komen Breast Cancer Foundation, which has become the nation's leading catalyst in the fight against breast cancer. Anybody who wonders if one person can make a difference need look no farther than Nancy Brinker's crusade for the answer.

Cancer is something we never expect will happen to us. Unlike the major events in our lives—weddings, graduations, and the birth of children—most of us are unprepared to deal with the traumatic impact of being diagnosed with this disease. Suzy Komen and Nancy Brinker didn't expect breast cancer any more than I did. But if you have been diagnosed or someone you care about is fighting this disease, *Winning the Race* gives you an advantage we never had—an easy-to-read source of inspiration and access to crucial information that can help you through this difficult time. This book and the many services the wonderful and dedicated people of the Komen Foundation provide can be a Godsend when facing the fight of your life.

I like to think of my diagnosis date as September 26, 1974 "B.K"—Before Komen; before Nancy made her promise to Suzy to end breast cancer as a life-threatening disease. Before she made a world without breast cancer her life's work and took to the streets of America with the Komen Race for the Cure Series®. Before the Susan G. Komen Breast Cancer Foundation raised millions of dollars to fund cutting-edge research that has given us breakthrough therapies to fight this insidious disease. And long before the Komen Foundation's crucial education, screening and treatment programs helped to save the lives of thousands of women across this country.

Nancy and I, like most breast cancer survivors, celebrate life every day. And in 2002, the Komen Foundation has something special to celebrate, too—twenty years of taking its message of hope "out of the shadows and into the streets." From the suburbs to the cities. From corporate boardrooms to community clinics. From the halls of medicine to the halls of Congress. And in doing so, it has truly changed the world.

A few years ago, I was privileged to attend the dedication of a new hospital devoted to cancer care. As I sat on the dais waiting for my turn to speak, I glanced at the program and read a poem I have never forgotten:

Hope is the thing with feathers
That perches in the soul
And sings that tune without words
And never stops at all.

The words are Emily Dickinson's, but the message is pure Nancy Brinker. I hope you will read this extraordinary book; learn from it; and live for yourself and the ones you love.

Take it from one who knows: "The race is won one step at a time." The first step is to take charge of your life and your care.

Betty Ford
Former First Lady of the United States

Acknowledgements

More than twenty years have passed since a simple promise between two sisters became an international movement. The Susan G. Komen Breast Cancer Foundation and its mission to eradicate breast cancer have been my life's work and have become the passion of literally thousands of people across this country. I am proud of the progress we have made in our fight against this terrible disease. The breakthroughs have been remarkable, and I marvel every day at how far we have come on our journey.

As I sat at my desk working on this special Twentieth Anniversary edition, I reflected on the medical and educational advances we have made. But, I also found myself remembering the people I have met along the way—survivors, grieving families, physicians and researchers, and, of course, the volunteers. Their dedication to this cause has inspired me over the years and proven over and over again that we can all make a difference in our world.

There are so many to thank, it would take another book to do it properly. But I want to single out a few whose help on our mission and this book have been extraordinary.

First, I want to thank my partners in the promise. No one was more instrumental, did more, or cared more about making my promise to Suzy a reality than Norman Brinker. He never gave up on my dream, or me, and when I faced breast cancer myself, Norman was my anchor in the storm. There are few people in this world as special as Norman Brinker. My deepest thanks also go to the leadership and staff of the Komen Foundation, past and present. Susan Braun, our CEO, is a truly outstanding individual whose leadership and talent have made the Komen Foundation a model for philanthropic activism. We are lucky to have her at the helm.

Our current and former board members have given us wise counsel and direction to help guide our path. We couldn't have done it without them or our volunteer leaders across the country serving on 115 Komen boards. I want to also thank Linda Kay Peterson, our current chair, for her invaluable guidance and years of dedication, and Dr. LaSalle D. Leffall, Jr., for honoring us with his agreement to become the next Komen chair.

It is never easy to come up with the words to thank adequately a staff like the Komen Foundation's. For them, this isn't a job: It's a commitment of the heart. There isn't a more dedicated or talented group than the wonderful people of Komen, and I hope they know how much I appreciate their efforts every day. And, of course, I am also grateful to our corporate "angels" and our individual donors who have provided the crucial funds that support the Foundation's cutting-edge research, education, screening and treatment programs that have led to breakthroughs and saved lives.

This book has been a labor of love for so many, and I want to acknowledge their contributions as well. First, go many thanks to my terrific co-author, Chriss Winston, who helped me find just the right words to tell my story. With breast cancer research moving forward at a breakneck pace, keeping up with the medical and scientific progress isn't easy. But, this book must be as current as we can make it. Lives depend on it. So, thanks also go to Dr. Joyce O'Shaughnessy, Dr. George Peters, Dr. Fritz Barton, and Dr. John Bostwick for their contributions to this and earlier editions.

Our internal Komen review team spent untold hours fine-tuning every detail of the book: CEO Susan Braun; Andy Halpern, our general counsel; Diane Balma, our director of public policy and a survivor herself; and our director of communications, Susan Carter. And I want to say a special thank you to Sloane Burke-Baty, who did a remarkable job as our internal associate editor—juggling her editorial duties with her equally demanding responsibilities as manager of the Komen Race for the Cure Series.®

I also want to thank my assistant, Lori Capra, who keeps me on track and on time and whose patience and real commitment mean a great deal to me. And to my friend and colleague in this cause, Laurey Peat, I can only say how much I value her judgment, her humor, and her willingness always to tell me what I need to hear.

The words simply don't exist to tell my mother, Ellie, and my father, Marvin, how much I love them and appreciate all that they have done for me personally and for the Komen Foundation. They have been my tower of strength and my comfort and just saying "thank you" never seems enough for a lifetime of love. My family has always been my strength, and I also want to thank my cousins—Cindy Solls and her son Jack, Nancy and Mark Solls, and their children, Rob, Michelle, and Jessica.

I have been privileged to know and be treated by a number of tremendously talented physicians over the years. I want to especially acknowledge Dr. Fred Ames, Dr. Phil Evans, Dr. Taylor Wharton, Dr. Morris Fogelman, Dr. David A. Hidalgo, Dr. Rod Rohrich, and Dr. Steven Harms for their skill, their honesty, and their kindness. There is also a special place in my heart for Dr. George Blumenschein, who was both Suzy's physician and mine. But he is so much more. Dr. Blumenschein has also been my mentor and good friend who will never know how much he has meant to me over the years.

So many people have been a part of this book and my life just as so many have been a part of keeping my promise to Suzy over the past twenty years. We have come so far since we began the Komen Foundation. So many lives have been changed and saved—mine among them. Thank you to everyone who has cared enough to get involved.

About the Authors

ABOUT NANCY BRINKER

Before Nancy Brinker's sister, Suzy, died of breast cancer at the age of thirty-six, Nancy promised her that she would help others confronted with the disease that had devastated Suzy's young life. In 1982, Nancy founded the Susan G. Komen Breast Cancer Foundation in her sister's memory. Today the Foundation is a leader in the fight against breast cancer, advancing research, education, screening and treatment. By its twentieth birthday, the Foundation will have raised more than $400 million in the fight against this disease and funded more than 583 international grants.

Nancy established the Komen Race for the Cure® Series in 1983 in Dallas, Texas. Since that time, the Komen Race for the Cure® has grown from one local Race to the largest series of 5K runs and fitness walks in the world. The Komen Race for the Cure® Series has raised significant funds for education and outreach programs in more than 100 local communities across the country. In addition, the Race Series provides funding for leading-edge scientific research in the field of breast cancer.

Nancy Brinker is one of the most highly respected breast cancer patient advocates in the country. She has earned an international reputation over the past two decades for her courageous groundbreaking efforts to raise awareness and funding for women's health issues, particularly breast cancer.

In 1986, President Ronald Reagan appointed Nancy as one of only six laypersons to the prestigious National Cancer Advisory Board. She served under both President Reagan and President George Herbert Walker Bush in this capacity. In 1991, Vice President Dan Quayle appointed her to the three-member President's Cancer Panel. In 1992, she chaired the Subcommittee on Breast Cancer.

Nancy has served on the Board of Directors of the Susan G. Komen Breast Cancer Foundation; Manpower, Inc.; U.S. Oncology, Inc.; and Harvard University's Center for Cancer Prevention as well as a number of advisory boards including the Fred Hutchinson Cancer Research Center and the University of Texas M. D. Anderson Cancer Center. She has also been a consultant to Astra-Zeneca Pharmaceuticals for Breast Cancer Awareness Month.

In May 2001, Nancy's strength as a leader was recognized by President George W. Bush when he appointed her to the prestigious post of United States ambassador to Hungary.

As a breast cancer survivor herself, Nancy has testified before Congress on major breast cancer and healthcare issues from the need for increased cancer research funding to barriers to clinical trials and has appeared on most major television news programs as a leader in the fight against breast cancer. She has spoken at major international medical and public health seminars and conferences on breast cancer issues.

Nancy has received numerous awards for her work in the field of breast cancer, including:

> ❧ *Ladies' Home Journal* 100 Most Important Women of the 20th Century and the "Champions of Women's Health Award"
> ❧ *Biography Magazine's* 25 Most Powerful Women in America
> ❧ National Foundation for the Center for Disease Control "Champion of Prevention" Award
> ❧ *Prevention Magazine* Hall of Fame: "They Changed Your Life" Award
> ❧ American Society of Clinical Oncologists 2000 Special Recognition Award
> ❧ Sisters' Network 2001 Lifetime Achievement Award

- ℜ Salomon Smith Barney Extraordinary Achievement Award
- ℜ Cancer Survivors Hall of Fame
- ℜ The 2001 Global Conference Institute "Healthcare Humanitarian Award"
- ℜ Cino del Duca Award, Xth International Congress on Anticancer Therapy, Paris
- ℜ Treaty of Paris Signatory, World Summit on Cancer, Paris
- ℜ Texas Governor's Award for Outstanding National Service
- ℜ Vincent T. Lombardi Cancer Center Symbol of Caring Award
- ℜ Layman's Award of the Society of Surgical Oncology
- ℜ Fox Chase Cancer Center Reimann Honor Award
- ℜ Hadassah Myrtle Wreath Award
- ℜ University of Illinois Distinguished Alumni Award and Alumni Achievement Award
- ℜ Albert Einstein College of Medicine Lizette H. Sarnoff Award for Volunteer Services
- ℜ National Association of Women's Health Professionals Special Services Award

Nancy has a terrific extended family including her son Eric; her parents and cousins; her late sister Suzy's husband, Stan, and their children, Stephanie and Scott; and the latest addition to the Komen family—Suzy's granddaughter, Maddie. Her home remains in Palm Beach, Florida.

ABOUT CHRISS WINSTON

Chriss Winston was the first woman to serve as chief White House speechwriter. A Washington communications veteran of both the Reagan and first Bush administrations, she is now a freelance writer whose work appears in many nationally known publications. Chriss lives with her husband and son in Pomfret, Maryland.

Introduction

"You've got a friend."
Carole King

"It's a girl!" Her name is Susan Madeline Komen, and she was born on March 14, 2000, to the delight of her proud parents and grandfather, happy great-grandparents, and absolutely thrilled aunt—me. But there is someone missing in Maddie's young life. There should be a loving grandmother cheering the arrival of this beautiful baby with her father's eyes and happy disposition. Maddie Komen is my sister Suzy's first grandchild. She's a precious little girl who would have been the apple of her grandmother's eye. Would have been. But little Madeline will never be held by her grandmother. Suzy won't teach her how to be a lady as she tried to teach me or show her how to sit a horse or tell her wonderful stories about growing up in Peoria.

Susan Goodman Komen died of breast cancer on August 4, 1980. She was 36 years old and my best friend. Suzy would have loved Maddie, and Maddie would have loved her. But breast cancer took Suzy from us—neither quickly nor quietly, and without warning or reason. Twenty-two years later, I still miss her.

Suzy and I each had our dreams. They were as different as we were, but on one thing we completely agreed; that we would always be there for each other. As girls, the two of us had already mapped out much of our lives. We would take care of our parents together when the time came, share a

1

room in the old folks' home one day, and compare stories about our husbands, kids and grandchildren.

It never dawned on me that things could turn out so differently. No, breast cancer was the last thing either of us expected to devastate both our lives. Even I, with the most vivid of imaginations, never thought about what it would be like to spend three years watching this disease slowly and painfully suck the life out of my best friend. Not once did I fantasize about what it would be like to hear those dreaded words, "It's cancer," spoken about me. Nor did I think for a minute that I'd start an international foundation for breast cancer research, education, screening and treatment in my sister's memory.

But what we could not imagine then became the reality of our lives later. The year was 1977 when Suzy was diagnosed with breast cancer. She died three years later after a long and difficult battle. I began the Susan G. Komen Breast Cancer Foundation in 1982 and was diagnosed with breast cancer myself in 1984. This book celebrates what have been twenty amazing years of pain and progress; fear and faith; and most of all hope that one day Suzy's dream, of a world where no woman will have to suffer as she did, would come true. It was this dream that became my promise to her.

This book is part biography, part autobiography, and part breast health manual, but I want it to be something more than that. I want it to be a good friend to any and all who read it. When you are first diagnosed with breast cancer, your world is shattered. Panic is the most common reaction, followed quickly by rage and depression and a terrible feeling of helplessness. When that happens, you need a friend who will comfort you, teach you and inspire you; someone who will boost your spirits and keep *you* on the right track; someone who will always tell you the truth no matter what.

I wrote this book to be that friend to you or to someone you care about. Friends tell each other the whole story—the good and the bad, and that's what I've tried to do here, too. I've told you what happened to Suzy. The story is painful at times. It certainly was painful to write. Then I've told you my own story with its very different outcome. Suzy and I fought our illnesses in two totally different ways, medically and mentally. I hope you will learn from both our stories.

I've also told you about the Komen Foundation and the struggle to make it what it is today. And finally, the book seeks to empower you by giving you a head start with important breast cancer information. There's a lot to learn about breast health that most of us never got in school. This book tries to give you the information to take charge of your own breast health and care, if need be. Just understanding breast cancer won't prevent it, but it will make the road considerably easier—at least easier to follow.

My object isn't to frighten you with stories of awful treatments or scary statistics on breast cancer—quite the contrary. Suzy was frightened: so frightened that her fear paralyzed her judgment. She is gone, and all the information in the world might not have saved her in the end. But I believe, in my heart, that had all of us been better informed about breast cancer, had we known enough to try every option available, her life might have been prolonged if not saved.

I have learned a great deal over the years, first as the sister of a breast cancer patient, then as the patient myself, and finally as a patient advocate. Through it all my family has always been there for me; helping me learn; helping me cope; keeping my head out of the clouds and my feet on the ground; and most of all just loving me.

So, I'd like to try and be there for you even if it's just for the few hours you read this book. I want you to be healthy. To take charge of your own breast health and care. I want you to live. So, let me share with you, in this and the chapters to follow, what I've learned over the last two decades about taking charge of your life and your care.

When I was struggling to find a way to keep my promise to Suzy to do something about breast cancer, the first thing I realized was that I was woefully undereducated when it came to really understanding this disease. So, I hit the books, and what I learned really shocked me. Remember, at that time, the pain of Vietnam was still fresh, and my initial research revealed some startling numbers. I learned that 59,000 Americans had died in that costly war. It was a terrible loss for our country and for so many families whose husbands and sons and a few daughters didn't come home. But then, I discovered that 339,000 American women died of breast cancer during that same time. I was outraged. No one protested *their* loss; no one spoke up for *these* women—these wives, mothers, daughters, and sisters. That silence became my cause; and, in 1982, the cause became the Susan G. Komen Breast Cancer Foundation. I had found the way to keep my promise to Suzy.

I recruited a small group of close friends, some of whom had personal experiences with breast cancer, and we set off on a journey that most people thought was quixotic at best. The truth was, we didn't know any better. It didn't take us long to realize, however, that if we were going to have any hope of achieving our goal—the end of breast cancer—we had to change two crucial environments: one, cultural and the other clinical. That was a tough assignment. In those days, in the early 80s, people were afraid to talk about cancer. Most wouldn't even use the word. Neither would the media. People called it the "Big C." It's hard for us to imagine it now, twenty years later; but back then, thousands of women were dying of breast cancer every year and many thousands more were being diagnosed, and we weren't supposed to talk about it.

Eventually, I came to think of breast cancer as the "Silent Epidemic." I became convinced that the only way to win the battle against this disease was to break the silence—to shout our message loud enough and long enough so that we simply could not be ignored by our government, our physicians or the research community any longer. We were a pretty noisy bunch and proud of it.

Helen Keller, a hero of mine, said, "The most pathetic person in the world is someone who has sight, but has no vision." To get beyond the fear with a message of hope became Komen's vision. Thanks to the efforts of so many, we have come a long way on our journey to create a world without breast cancer. Today, words like *mammogram* and *breast health* that were rarely heard twenty years ago are now dinner table conversation.

Every day, I see signs of progress all around us when a woman passes me by on the street wearing a pink Komen Race for the Cure® survivor T-shirt, or when the results of a clinical trial bring new hope. And I hear our progress, too, when a talk show host or the network news takes up our fight, and I feel it deep inside when major corporations, who once upon a time would not open their doors to me, now embrace our cause with the wonderful passion of the converted.

I see our progress in the statistics, too. When we began Komen in the early 80s, the mortality rate for breast cancer was growing. In 2001, the Public Health Service announced that breast cancer death rates declined an average of 3.4 percent between 1995 and 1998. That's more than double the rate of decline while

TAKING CHARGE OF BREAST CANCER

breakthroughs in detection and treatment are increasing at an astonishing rate. There's a reason. Before Komen and the breast cancer movement, Washington put little focus on this terrible disease. At Komen, we soon learned that there is power in numbers, and as the crowds grew in Komen Races for the Cure® across America, politicians began to take notice that there was a new "movement" in town. In the early 80s, the federal government spent less than $35 million a year on breast cancer research. In the Bush Administration's 2002 budget, federal funding for breast cancer research, prevention, screening and education programs reached *$766 million dollars.* Volunteers of the Komen Foundation helped apply the pressure that changed the priorities in Washington. For twenty years, Komen's "angels," as I like to call them, have set the pace for winning the race. We've been fundraisers and cheerleaders. We've had to break new ground and a few eggs along the way to do it. We've held seminars, and screening sessions, and Races, and more than a few hands along the way, too. We've worn out more sneakers than we can count, but we made all those blisters and sore muscles count for something important. The dollars and the awareness we raised have helped thousands of women in their personal battles with breast cancer. Who knows how many lives Komen's education, screening and treatment programs have saved? We've come a long way. It's been quite a journey, but the journey isn't over. The race isn't won—yet.

I have learned so much over the years about breast cancer, about creating an organization out of nothing; and making a difference. But, in facing my own breast cancer, I learned some things that I couldn't find in a book, but I wished I had. So, I want to share what I've learned about living with breast cancer with you, too—what I call my Seven Lessons for Life so that when you finish reading this book, you can take charge of your life and your care should that day come. Nothing is more important. Most of these lessons will be expanded on later but for now, they're a great "To Do" list to keep on your fridge or your bedroom mirror.

LESSON NUMBER 1
BE YOUR OWN BEST FRIEND

When you face a serious illness, your spouse, your mother, your golfing buddy, your aerobics instructor, even your poodle can all help; but you must be your own very best friend. You've got to take charge of your life, and the best way to do that is to become an expert on your own illness.

It's called patient empowerment. Twenty years ago, when Suzy was diagnosed, it wasn't even in our vocabulary, but it's a whole new world today. You may have heard about the woman doctor isolated at a research station in Antarctica who found a lump in her breast. Because of the severe weather, she couldn't be evacuated for treatment for several months, but this was a woman who wouldn't wait.

She took matters into her own hands. In an amazing rescue mission, the U.S. Air Force airdropped crucial medicine and state-of-the-art equipment to her. Thanks to new technology, she could talk directly with physicians stateside about her care and send test results digitally for a more accurate diagnosis. She's still alive and well as I write this; this woman gave herself the best possible chance by taking charge of her own care. You should, too.

Today, technology can give *you* power through access to crucial information that was once only the province of physicians. But like the Antarctic researcher, don't rely on someone else to do your homework. Read.

Watch television. Surf the Net. The Internet is an information jackpot for folks like us. You can find reports on the latest clinical trials and breakthroughs in research and treatment. You can connect with other survivors or even talk to physicians in medical chat rooms. The resource section at the back of this book lists some of the best sources of Internet information. But a word of warning: always be careful and discriminate about the information you receive on the Internet. Avoid on-line diagnoses or con-

"It's a part of the cure, to wish to be cured."

Seneca

tent that is undocumented, undated, or without peer review, and consult with your medical provider before making any decision concerning your breast health or breast cancer treatment.

With a little caution and good sense, you can use all these sources to find options; to understand what tests you must take; which ones you're going to have to pay for and what's involved; and connect with others facing the same fight. In other words, maximize all the wonderful resources out there today to take charge of your own care.

LESSON NUMBER 2
BE YOUR PHYSICIAN'S COLLEAGUE

One of the side effects, so to speak, of the patient empowerment movement has been a dramatic change in the patient/physician relationship. You should expect more from your physician today, especially more respect. You've got a brain, and your physician should understand that. You've also got important information about your care, how you feel physically and emotionally, that your physician should consider. Too many medical providers today still give little or no validity to their patients' perspectives or insights that could prove invaluable.

If you've got information you believe your physician needs, don't wait to be asked. Tell him or her immediately. If the response you get goes something like, "You've been reading too much," or "Stay off the Internet," maybe you've got the wrong physician.

LESSON NUMBER 3
DON'T LET YOUR BODY PUSH YOU AROUND

When you're battling a serious illness, depression and anger go with the territory, but attitude is everything. Ronald Reagan certainly knew that.

He once joked, "Since I came to the White House, I got two hearing aids, a colon operation, skin cancer, a prostate operation, and I was shot. The damn thing is I've never felt better in my life." What I've learned is that you've got to fight back. If you feel like a human time bomb—and everyone does at some point or another—cut the wires.

If that means you need to cry . . . then cry. If you want to vent, call a friend and vent. Understand your limitations and accept them. Sometimes winning is finishing a walk, or a treatment, or getting through one more day. And remember to laugh. It may be a cliché but that doesn't make it any less true—laughter *is* the best medicine.

Finally, don't underestimate the power of spirituality in recovery. We've all heard stories about inexplicable "cures"; people given weeks or months to live who defy the odds. I've known many over the past twenty years. The truth is we don't know how attitude impacts patient outcome. The brain and its power over disease is still an enigma in many ways.

> *"Humor is contagious. Laughter is infectious. Both are good for your health."*
> William Fry, M.D.

What we do know is that spirituality and prayer have historically been linked with the power to heal. With increasing public interest in complementary therapies, the research community is focusing new efforts involving the healing effects of prayer—a mystery that up to now has remained outside the realm of scientific understanding. By encouraging integration of complementary treatments with conventional medicine, we can treat the whole patient and improve healing.

Some people scoff at the notion of prayer-based or spiritual interventions, but today's knowledge wasn't achieved by calmly accepting the status quo. Taking charge of our own care sometimes means pushing the envelope and stepping forward into the unknown. If we rejected everything we don't understand, we would make very little progress in this world.

David Ben-Gurion, the father of Israel, said, "In order to be a realist, you've got to believe in miracles." I think that's pretty good advice.

LESSON NUMBER 4
YOU'VE GOT A FRIEND—LOTS OF THEM

Even though you must take charge of your care, you don't have to walk what can be a difficult path alone. Don't be afraid to ask for help.

I've already told you how important I believe family has been to my life, but the story of Chris and Stefanie Spielman is another story of inspiring love and sacrifice. In 1996, Chris Spielman was a linebacker with the Buffalo Bills when he suffered a terrible neck injury that sidelined him for the season. Some thought his career was over, but Chris never gave up. Just when he was ready to return to football he got some devastating news he didn't expect. His wife, Stefanie, was diagnosed with breast cancer. She would need a mastectomy and chemo-therapy, and that meant recovery time. With a four-year-old and a two-year-old at home, for Chris, the decision was easy. Football would have to wait. He took another year off to become a "pro-Dad" so Stefanie could concentrate on fighting her cancer.

That's what I call a real love story.

Families can be just what the doctor ordered, but don't forget, that's what friends are for, too. When you become ill, your first reaction may be, "I hate to ask." Ask! I've found most people want to help but are often unsure how to approach a friend with breast cancer. They don't want to intrude. They're afraid of saying or doing the wrong thing. Most want to do whatever you want them to do. Friends and family can make a huge difference. So help them help you.

LESSON NUMBER 5
KEEP YOUR DANCE CARD FULL

Stay busy. Set new goals for yourself. As Eleanor Roosevelt said, "Do the one thing that you think you can't do."

Go back to school. Join the local playhouse. Or take a hike. That's just what 17 breast cancer survivors did—I mean literally. These brave women, some who had just finished chemotherapy, climbed Mt. Aconcagua in Argentina, the highest peak in the Western Hemisphere—nearly 23,000 feet. That hike became "Expedition Inspiration," an organization that sponsors climbs around the world to benefit breast cancer research.

These women were determined to prove that cancer would not slow them down, and it didn't. Not all of us could or should undertake that kind of physical activity, but each of us can try new things and challenge ourselves in ways that may change the outcome of our illness.

LESSON NUMBER 6
BE AN EVANGELIST FOR YOUR CAUSE

When I think of evangelists, the first thing that comes to my mind is a picture of thousands of women walking and running in a sea of pink caps. They are breast cancer survivors joining in the Komen Race for the Cure® Series; and they are true evangelists in the breast cancer movement.

Over a million people participate in the Komen Race for the Cure® every year raising millions of dollars to support breast cancer programs, but they participate for different reasons. This is how one woman described her motivation. She said, "I run for those who have received their wings, and for those who have not yet found out ... for those who will have surgery, chemo, sickness and anger ... I run because I have been given the gift of life."

Not all Komen Race for the Cure® participants have breast cancer, but they are all evangelists for our cause. Not every evangelist races, however. Some participate in Bowl for the Cure,™ Sing for the Cure,™ and even Cook for the Cure™ events. Believe it or not, we've had couples getting married sign up wedding guests as teams in the race to raise money for local breast cancer programs—on their wedding day.

It's their way of fighting for our cause. You've got to fight, too. That means learning how to work the clinical system *and* the political system. And it means getting involved beyond your own care to help others who have not been empowered.

In July 1999, Lance Armstrong, the American cyclist, won the Tour de France, one of the most physically demanding sporting events in the world. But what made his story so remarkable was that Lance was diagnosed in 1996 with advanced testicular cancer that had spread to his abdomen, lungs and brain. Now (as of writing this book), after treatment, he's cancer free.

"I have a responsibility to tell my story, to encourage people to fight," he said after his win. "You have to believe. You have to want to live." I believe part of that fight is being an evangelist for your cause.

LESSON NUMBER 7
DON'T STOP THINKING ABOUT THE FUTURE

No one who has ever faced a life-threatening illness ever does, but some simple advice is worth repeating. Stay up on your health and stay alive. Technology is giving us new tools to detect disease earlier. Use them.

Know the screening tests that can keep you and your family healthy. Have a basic physical regularly to check blood pressure, cholesterol, blood count, and urine. Chest X rays *"Tomorrow is another day."* Scarlett O'Hara are important, especially for smokers. If there is a history of colorectal cancer in your family, get tested for it.

Heart disease often has few symptoms, so an electrocardiogram could save your life. Men, get beyond your phobia and have your prostate checked. Women, don't put off your annual pelvic exam with a Pap test and a mammogram. Live healthy and never stop thinking about tomorrow.

Now, you know the most important lessons I've learned over the past twenty years as a patient advocate. There is more to come in the pages that follow. I only wish I could send you directly to a chapter titled, "The Cure"; but, so far, there is no cure. There is hope, however. When breast cancer is detected in its earliest stages, there is a greater than 90 percent five-year survival rate. My cancer was detected early; my sister's wasn't. I had the opportunity to marshal my possibilities; my sister did not. I took charge of my care; Suzy left it to others. She was a product of her times and paid the ultimate price because of it, leaving behind two young children, a very lonely husband, two heartbroken parents, many wonderful friends . . . and me.

Through the Susan G. Komen Breast Cancer Foundation, I have been able to keep Suzy's memory alive. The women and men who have become cherished members of our cause have helped, each in his or her own way, to fill the vast void in my heart. It's difficult for me to imagine Suzy as a grandmother because she is forever frozen in time—a beautiful and loving thirty-six-year-old mother without a gray hair or a wrinkle, but also a woman who never got the chance to see her children grow up. And when I think I just can't do this another day, that is what drives me . . . my dream that no mother should ever again have to leave her children behind because of breast cancer.

Maddie will never know the wonderful woman who was my sister, but I believe in my heart of hearts that because of Suzy, because of the breast cancer movement and the work we do at Komen, Maddie and her generation will one day live in a world without the terrible fear of breast cancer. No grandmother ever left a more precious legacy.

The Komen Foundation has come a long way over the past twenty years. The journey is over for Suzy, but it isn't over for us. The race isn't won. But I know that just as we have shared the fight, one day, we will also share the victory.

Suzy didn't want anyone to suffer the way she did. I don't either. The good news is . . . you might not have to.

Chapter One
Suzy's Story

"A sister is both your mirror and your opposite."
Elizabeth Fishel

The first time I can remember hearing the words *breast cancer* was back in 1956, which seems like a lifetime ago, now. In that era of "I Like Ike" and Elvis Presley, I was ten years old and living in Peoria, Illinois, with my parents, Eleanor and Marvin Goodman, and my older sister, Susan. Our home was on a quiet, tree-lined street in a peaceful neighborhood where every neighbor was a friend, much like a scene right out of *Father Knows Best*. It was a traditional life and the rules were clearly laid out. Dinner was served on a white tablecloth and good manners were mandatory. Mealtime was family time in the Goodman household and that meant no interruptions. No boyfriends, no phone calls—no nothing. Dad was the family leader and authoritarian, of that there was no doubt. Although we always felt loved, he was a very strict man who demanded respect. It was that discipline that gave us our structure and me my drive. To some, our childhood might seem a little old-fashioned now, but that kind of loving home where children are challenged to be their best never goes out of style.

It would hurt Dad's feelings terribly if I said I thought he loved Suzy more, but their relationship *was* different. Suzy was his first child and born a bit premature. She was a meeker and milder child, not to mention a lot smaller than me. He idolized little Suzy; and in his eyes, she could do no wrong. The truth of the matter is, she *did* no wrong. I, on the other hand, started out on the wrong foot from the beginning. I was supposed to be a boy. I weighed in at over a hundred pounds in second grade and had all the grace and poise of a baby elephant. I wasn't as cuddly as my sister, but I had a quick, curious mind. Dad simply expected more from me. Looking back now, I'm grateful for being taught to push harder, but back then it was sometimes hard to swallow.

My mother, on the other hand, has always been a woman of amazing patience, kindness, and inner strength. She allowed my father to "run" the family, yet she was the one who knew all our secrets, kept all our confidences. When something needed to be done, we depended on her for results. And she never let us down. Mom was a great mediator between my father and everyone else. Her secret weapon was humor, and even in an argument, she could manage to get a smile from my father. She was and still is the world's best peacekeeper. That was perhaps my mother's most useful gift to us—her ability to find the humor in any situation. She can still make me laugh at myself and the world around me.

But what has truly defined Mom has always been her willingness to help others. Without a doubt, she has earned the title of "volunteer extraordinaire" ten times over. In fact, when we were growing up, unlike most of her friends, she didn't play bridge. It wasn't that she didn't know how to play, she just thought there were more important things she could do with her life. She ran the Girl Scouts in Peoria, was a tireless charity volunteer for what seemed like a thousand causes, and never missed a PTA meeting. Mom taught Suzy and me that each of us

has a responsibility to care for those around us. It is difficult to imagine anyone more caring and involved in their
community than my mother. Yet, she was usually in the
kitchen baking cookies when Suzy and I came home from
school and always had dinner waiting for my father at the
end of each day. And she did it all with a smile on her face.

Suzy and I were unable to suppress squeals of joy
when we were informed one night at dinner that we were
going to visit our favorite aunt, Rose, all the way in New
York City. Since Suzy was thirteen, Mom and Dad felt
we were old enough to make the trip by plane to the big
city by ourselves. To me, it was to be an exciting adventure (never mind the fact that our parents would put us
safely on the plane and Aunt Rose would be waiting at
the other end to pick us up).

That night after dinner my mother came into our
bedroom while we were dutifully doing our homework
and told us she had something to talk to us about. She
wanted to remind us that although Aunt Rose was feeling great and looked good she had been very sick with
breast cancer and had an operation called a mastectomy.
Suzy quickly jumped in and told Mom we both knew
about the operation and she didn't need to explain the
details of Aunt Rose's surgery. In the back of my mind I
had an idea what a mastectomy was, but I could tell, even
then, that the subject was uncomfortable for Suzy—so I
didn't ask any questions. Any subject with even so much
as a hint of violence, pain, or mutilation would upset her
terribly. I remember when Suzy's stallion was being
gelded, she ran away screaming with her hands over her
face while I sat up in a nearby tree and, although I winced
and covered my eyes, through parted fingers I watched
the whole thing with great interest.

By the time we saw Aunt Rose, so ebullient and full
of life, laughing and flirting with her new husband (her

fourth), all thoughts that she had once been sick passed completely from our minds. We listened intently while Rose told of her exotic safari in Africa. Oh, how I admired this woman. She did anything she wanted to, any time she wanted to do it. She was independent and free-spirited, and I wanted to be just like her. Suzy admired her too, but for different reasons. She saw in Aunt Rose the epitome of femininity. And she was right. Aunt Rose was truly glamorous. She entered and exited every room just like Loretta Young, with a chiffon scarf floating through the air. Her clothes were always beautiful and her perfume wafted behind her in a way that left her on your mind long after she was gone. And did she have a way with men! She knew how to get men to do anything and everything she wanted them to do, and she did it by making those men feel as if they were the most important and wonderful thing in her life.

On our third night in New York, something happened that would have a lasting effect on Suzy and me. Aunt Rose had taken us shopping, skating, and to the theater. We had had a long day, and Suzy and I were simply exhausted. As sometimes happens when two sisters are both tired, we got into a little squabble before bedtime. Whatever the argument was about we just couldn't seem to resolve it between ourselves this time, so Suzy marched in to discuss the matter with Aunt Rose. All of a sudden Suzy came tearing back into our room in a hysterical frenzy. I had never seen her so upset. She looked terrified. When I finally got her to calm down long enough to tell me what was wrong, she reported that she had gone into Aunt Rose's room without knocking and had accidentally seen the scars on her chest. She said they were terribly gruesome and she couldn't understand how Aunt Rose had lived through such mutilation. Naturally, I had to check out the situation for myself. So I tiptoed

back to Aunt Rose's room and quietly opened the door
to get a quick peek. Well, Suzy wasn't kidding. Not only
were the scars severe, but her chest looked concave and
burned from high-voltage cobalt treatments. I could
even faintly see her heart beating through thin, purple
skin. Aunt Rose had had what is known as a Halsted radical mastectomy on her left side. Although the procedure
is rarely done today, it was considered common treatment for breast cancer for nearly a hundred years and
was certainly common back then in 1956. The Halsted
radical removes not only the breast but all the underarm
lymph nodes, the chest muscles, and some additional fat
and skin. The truth is, her particular operation *was* unat-
tractive. I have since learned more about the procedure
and realize that hers was poorly done. But, as I softly
closed the door and began to walk back to Suzy, I heard
Aunt Rose singing happily to her husband. I decided
Aunt Rose didn't need my sympathy. Aunt Rose was living a fuller, richer, more exciting life than anyone else I
knew. If her mastectomy didn't bother her, why should
it bother me? But Suzy never got over it. The memory of
Aunt Rose's chest haunted her forever.

One of my favorite "boys," little Linus of *Peanuts*
fame, says that "Sisters are the crabgrass in the lawn of
life." Not my sister! As we got older, Suzy and I became
just about as close as two sisters can get. I thought she
was perfect. Suzy was beautiful, kind, and loving, not
only to me but to everyone. There was a goodness and
gentleness about my sister that went unnoticed by no
one. She was the star of our hometown of Peoria, the
high school homecoming queen, the college beauty
queen. She was everyone's darling, and I don't think
there was a soul who ever met her who didn't fall in love
with her—men, women, and children alike. This was the
era of Grace Kelly's fairytale marriage to Prince Ranier,

and I was convinced that a handsome prince one day would, no doubt, sweep Suzy off her feet, and I suppose I secretly hoped there might be an extra one there for me, too. I worshipped Suzy and used to follow her around everywhere. She never seemed to mind. If she did, she never showed it. I, on the other hand, was bigger, heavier, and taller than most of my friends *and* her friends. I developed my own way of getting attention. I was a tomboy and a mischief-maker and delighted in nothing more than spending hours galloping around on horseback. Suzy tried desperately to teach me about all the pretty things in life: how to fix my hair, apply makeup, and coordinate my wardrobe. None of it seemed to work. I was still a big, sort of clumsy girl with two left feet. The boys didn't know I was alive, except that I was Susan Goodman's younger sister, the one with her nose always buried in a book. It was beginning to look like my future would be limited to frogs, not princes. The only frustration we ever had with each other was that it bothered me that Suzy seemed content to stay right where she was just as it bothered her to constantly see the discontent in my eyes.

Suzy came back to Peoria after she graduated from college and got a job modeling locally. Eventually, she married her college sweetheart, Stan Komen, who while not technically a prince, was and is a wonderful man. Stan and Suzy had a very good marriage. Although they were unable to have children of their own, they soon adopted two beautiful babies, Scott and Stephanie. Suzy had everything she wanted: a loving husband and a family of her own.

College, for me, was the first time I felt I belonged anywhere. At the University of Illinois, the baby fat came off and so did the braces, thank God. I was active in many school projects and finally began to have confidence in myself. I felt independent and responsible and ready to take on the world. After graduating, I packed up my bags and moved to Dallas, home of my father's older sister, Aunt Ruth. As a child, I had spent many vacations in Texas and often dreamed of one day living on the wide-open ranchland I had come to love. That way, I figured I hadn't spent all those years learning how to ride for nothing. When Dad finally agreed to the move, or at least realized he couldn't stop me, he made it clear that I would have to support myself, and I knew I couldn't do that on horseback.

So I walked into Neiman-Marcus and told the personnel director my situation. "Look," I said, "my parents are not happy about my being in Texas. I need a job, and I need a good one." I started as an executive trainee and worked up to an assistant couture buyer. More importantly, I was lucky enough to learn the art of marketing and public relations from one of the masters—Stanley Marcus himself. It was at Neiman-Marcus that I also met my first husband. The marriage was troubled, but it produced a wonderful miracle—my son, Eric.

Although we were hundreds of miles apart, Suzy and I spoke every day by phone. Our daily conversations were something I grew to depend on and cherish. She kept me up-to-date on what was happening in Peoria and I filled her in on my life in Dallas. We discussed our children, our husbands, and our careers at great length. Suzy's calm, kind-hearted way was a perfect contrast to my frantic, impatient nature. In a way, I was her third child and she was my second mother. Above all, we made each other laugh.

It was about this time that Suzy and I became aware we both had a common and non-threatening condition called fibrocystic disease. This is a lumpiness in the breast caused by the breast's response to hormonal levels as they change from month to month. Lumpy, or cystic, breasts are often accompanied by pain or tenderness that fluctuates with the menstrual cycle, becoming more noticeable and painful just before your period begins. Fibrocystic breasts is by far the most common breast disorder, and nearly all women's breasts develop some degree of this condition at one time or another. We will talk about fibrocystic breasts in more detail in chapter 4, but the point I want to make now is that neither Suzy nor I was concerned in the least about our condition. Occasionally, Suzy's physician would perform what is called a needle aspiration. Using a needle and syringe to withdraw fluid or a small amount of tissue from a breast lump can show whether that lump is a fluid-filled cyst or a solid mass. Suzy's lumps were fluid-filled cysts. The procedure was nothing that caused her alarm. Our physicians assured us that eight out of ten lumps were not dangerous in any way and that we had nothing to worry about. Besides, we both felt young and invincible.

Although it has been more than twenty years, I can remember the phone call I received from Suzy one Tuesday afternoon as if it were yesterday. Her physician had found a lump that was not a cyst. He recommended a biopsy. A biopsy is the surgical removal and microscopic examination of tissue to see if cancer cells are present. Now, you must understand that my sister was the most nurturing, loving woman in the world. She took it upon herself to help everyone who crossed her path. And, by force of habit, we not only allowed her to comfort us when we needed it, we grew to depend on it. Hearing uneasiness in her voice, as much as she tried to hide it, was unnatural. She didn't sound like herself, and it frightened me. Of course, my parents and I tried to make light of the situation and tell Suzy we were sure that everything would be fine. But, to be honest, we weren't sure at all. Not at all. And although none of us mentioned it, the memory of

our visit with Aunt Rose so many years before came back
to life vividly in all our minds.

I decided to fly home to Peoria. Suzy said it wasn't
necessary, that she would call me when they found out
the results. I insisted on coming anyway, saying I wanted
to be there for the celebration when the tests came back
negative. But when I got off the plane, my father was
waiting there alone with an expression on his face I will
never forget. He didn't have to say a word. *At the age of
thirty-three, Suzy had breast cancer.* What happened from
this point on is still difficult for me to talk about because
I am so much more knowledgeable on the subject today.
*If I had only known then what I know now and what you
will know when you finish this book.*

The truth of the matter is that growing up in the
small town of Peoria, our family had been treated our
whole lives by one physician. He was a nice man and a
fine physician, and we relied on him for all of our childhood illnesses. He was probably the last of his kind, an
older physician who still made house calls and was a
friend not only to us, but to everyone he treated. Suzy
trusted him with her cancer the same way she trusted
him with her measles. This was the first of several mistakes Suzy might not have made if we had been better
educated about her disease. None of us knew enough to
inquire about seeking information from a major cancer
center near our town or from a group of physicians associated with a cancer center. He was our doctor. Period.

The most difficult concept to grasp about cancer is
the fact that when it is first detected, the patient usually
feels just fine. There is rarely any pain associated with
breast cancer in its early stages. So when you are told
you've got a life-threatening disease, and the treatment
sounds more heinous than the thought of a little lump in
the breast, it is understandable that a woman uneducated

about cancer might opt for no treatment at all. Such was the case with Suzy. My sister was terrified, naturally, but adamant against having a mastectomy. She wasn't vain in a negative sense, but she enjoyed every part of being a woman. That included having breasts. Two of them.

Our family physician called in a surgeon to review Suzy's case. It is important, if you are to learn from our mistakes, that I tell you a little bit about this surgeon. He was very handsome, very suave, and seemed very self-confident. He told us that her cancer was medullary carcinoma, and there were no lymph nodes involved. I will go into more detail about this medical terminology later on, but briefly what I understood him to mean was that, in his opinion, her cancer had not spread or metastasized to other parts of her body. According to Suzy, this surgeon—I will refer to him as Dr. Smith (not his real name)—told Suzy he could cure her. Even the most respected cancer experts in the country (which Dr. Smith certainly was not) talk about recovery in terms of surviving cancer or remission. They refrain from using the word *cure* because cancer can recur.

But that, of course, is exactly what Suzy wanted to hear, and who could blame her? Like many women (and for that matter, men, too), Suzy was of the frame of mind that the doctor was always right. When Dr. Smith smiled at her and said everything would be fine, she believed him without question. Suzy really didn't want to know everything there was to know about the disease, she just wanted him to make her better. She wanted not to be frightened anymore; she wanted to look normal; and she wanted to go back to being a healthy wife and mother.

Dr. Smith suggested performing a subcutaneous mastectomy, a procedure in which the outside of the breast is left intact but an incision is made and the breast tissue is removed. He would then do an implant ten days later. She would be left with a small scar but no more cancer. Suzy felt it was her best option. She was not referred to an oncologist—a cancer specialist—for a second opinion. The year was 1977; and although cancer treatments weren't nearly as sophisticated as they are today, we wish she had been offered the chance to participate in a clinical trial at a comprehensive cancer center. A clinical trial is an experimental study conducted with cancer patients, usually to evaluate a new treatment. Each study is designed to answer specific scientific questions. A patient is randomly assigned to one of several treatments in order to measure the success of one therapy versus another. Participants in clinical trials always receive the best treatment available and, unlike with placebo studies, always receive therapy. We can thank clinical trials for much of the progress against breast cancer we benefit from today

In a trial, Suzy would have been part of a closely monitored study conducted by physicians at a comprehensive cancer center giving her a much better chance for success. The rest of us tried very hard among ourselves to figure out what was best for her. But we were certainly no experts. Suzy was very upset, and Stan wanted to keep her calm, so he went along with what she wanted. My mother instinctively had a lot of questions, but was afraid to push too hard, fearing Suzy might decide to do nothing rather than go for more intense treatment. My father was devastated and did not know where to turn or what to do. It was very sad. I, being the rebel, wanted Suzy to get out of Peoria and have a second opinion at a comprehensive cancer center. To me, both our family physician and Dr. Smith, while their intentions were good, lacked the sophistication and exposure that can only be found through years of concentrated study in a given field. Their attention had been too diversified, treating everything from chicken pox to appendicitis. These are normal and admirable credentials, but in my opinion, not good enough for my sister's condition at that time. I wanted Suzy to have the best, I wanted her to come to Texas. But she wanted to stay in Peoria where she was comfortable and loved. And that is exactly what she did.

After Suzy's surgery, my parents, Stan, and I were all at the hospital anxiously awaiting the results. Dr. Smith walked confidently in the room and said, "You can relax; we got it all. I believe she's cured." My heart sank because even then I knew enough to know that *cure* is a very difficult word to use in reference to cancer.

Let me set the record straight about Suzy's physicians: Neither of them had anything but good intentions, nor did they want anything less than good health for her. Both of these physicians did their best to save my sister's life. It wasn't good enough. But Suzy loved them. She felt that the better she knew her doctors, the closer the physician/patient relationship, the better the prognosis. She felt that because these doctors were her *friends*, they wouldn't let her down. They *couldn't* let her down because friends don't do that to each other.

Suzy, and maybe all of us, also suffered from something I call the "Oz Syndrome." Once upon a time, most of us looked upon our physicians much like Dorothy did the Wizard of Oz. In people's minds, physicians were all-powerful, all-knowing, nearly infallible beings in whose judgment we placed our unquestioning confidence and, sometimes, our lives. Over the past twenty years, that patient/physician relationship has changed as technology and the media have given patients access to information that allows them to make informed decisions on their own care. Like Oz, once the curtain was gone, once patients had been empowered, physicians could now be viewed for what they are—human beings who can be brilliant and kind, but who also can make mistakes. When Suzy was diagnosed, most people didn't question the advice of their physicians.

In Suzy's case, aside from radiation, I don't remember any other treatment or adjuvant therapy being suggested. Nowadays it is common to perform additional tests such as lymph node dissections or sentinal node biopsies, bone marrow analyses, bone scans, liver scans, or CAT scans to determine whether the cancer has metastasized. And for many patients, chemotherapy and or hormonal therapy follow surgery. But Suzy had none of these.

For the next five months or so, Suzy felt pretty good. She was convinced she was cured. When I suggested she get a second opinion just to be sure, she became very sensitive. After all, her physician had told her she was fine. I was back in Dallas, having my own problems dealing with a failing marriage. Suzy didn't want to talk about her illness, so, God bless her, she spent hours on the phone each day counseling me. I was concerned because Suzy had a shallow cough that wouldn't go away and she really didn't seem to have her energy back. She was cheerful and happy, but that old zing and sparkle just wasn't there. I didn't dare suggest that she was still sick. How could I, when Suzy was so optimistic? Quietly, I worried.

Before six months had gone by, our worst nightmare became a reality. Suzy found another lump. This time it was under her arm. Despite everyone's optimism, her cancer had spread.

I wanted to take Suzy to the M. D. Anderson Cancer Center in Houston because, through my contacts in Dallas, I had learned this facility was one of the best comprehensive cancer centers in the country. Suzy wasn't familiar with M.D. Anderson but she knew about the Mayo Clinic, so that's where she went next. It was at the Mayo clinic that we learned that her cancer had metastasized, or spread, to her lung and under her arm. There was a tumor the size of a quarter in the upper part of her right lung and suspicious shadows elsewhere on her chest X ray. Their recommendation was thirty days of radiation and then to "watch it." Well I, for one, was tired of "watching." I wanted to see some positive results.

Terror, rage, sadness, and above all, a feeling of complete and utter helplessness invaded me. Why was this happening to Suzy, of all people? What had she ever done to deserve to be so sick and so frightened? Although no one said anything aloud, we all knew my sister was now fighting for her life. *And it all happened so quickly.* She tried to keep up a brave front and would often talk of plans for the future, especially with Scott, only six, and Stephanie, just three—too small really to understand what was happening to their mother.

A major inspiration in Suzy's struggle for survival came from a surprising source: The former first lady of the United States, Betty Ford. In 1974, Mrs. Ford had told the world she had breast cancer. The whole country was shocked with the news of her cancer and mastectomy. The memory of her courage touched Suzy in a way that none of us could possibly understand because we hadn't gone through it ourselves. In Betty Ford, my sister found new strength. "Nan," she said, "if Mrs. Ford could admit she had breast cancer and tell the whole world she intended to fight it, well, then so can I." It wasn't the last time that Betty Ford would come to the rescue of the Goodman girls. The physicians at Mayo suggested Suzy have radiation therapy, which is a treatment using high-energy rays to damage cancer cells and stop them from growing. She did have the radiation, but it was not successful in slowing her disease. The cancer was out of control and there wasn't a damn thing we could do about it. But we had to try. Thank goodness, Suzy's plastic surgeon in Peoria suggested she try M. D.

Anderson. I guess there is something about hearing advice from a non-family member that allows it to sink in. It didn't matter; I was thrilled she had decided to give Houston a try.

Through contacts I had made when helping with a charity benefit for M. D. Anderson, I was able to get Suzy an appointment with an oncologist (a physician who specializes in the treatment of cancer) by the name of George Blumenschein. It is probably unfair for me to single out one man when there were so many men and women who tried desperately to save my sister's life. But Dr. Blumenschein represented an attitude and spirit in medicine that we had not seen up until this point. Before coming to M. D. Anderson, Suzy's treatment had always been determined by a single physician. Now, for the first time, Suzy was part of a team. *Dr. Blumenschein and his associates made Suzy a partner in every decision.* They were completely and totally honest with her and all of us about her condition. When Suzy arrived in Houston, she was a Stage 4 cancer patient. This means that the disease had spread to other organs in her body and was still growing. (You'll learn more about staging in chapter 6.) Stage 4 is a very critical situation. Dr. Blumenschein threw the book at her, in a sense. He not only told her everything, but he showed her the results of her tests. Rather than speak to Suzy in terms like "I will do this" or "I will do that," he said, "We can do this" or "Let's try that." He told Suzy exactly what her chances of survival were and what *they* had to do in order to fight this cancer. He said, "Susan, we will do everything we can to try to save you, but we can't do it without your help and cooperation." Suzy was not only allowed to ask questions, she was *encouraged* to do so. Dr. Blumenschein's approach to the disease was an aggressive one. After recommending removal of the lesion from her lung, he told Suzy that she had a 25 percent chance of survival, but that if she wouldn't give up, *he* wouldn't give up. He wanted to put her in a treatment protocol (that is, a specific course of therapy—in this case, a combination of drugs that was being tested in a clinical trial) at M. D. Anderson and promised her that if one didn't work he would try another. Thus began a saga of intense chemotherapy.

Chemotherapy is usually a combination of several highly-toxic drugs given together, delivered into the patient's bloodstream in an effort to kill fast-growing cells. The problem with chemotherapy is that it doesn't know the difference between the "good guys" and the "bad guys," so a lot of important healthy cells are killed in the process—including the cells of the mouth and stomach lining and hair roots. Depending on the drugs given, chemotherapy is often accompanied by nausea, mouth sores, hair thinning, and sometimes total hair loss. (Today, there are very effective drugs and other treatments that can relieve many of these side effects. See chapter 8.) Suzy experienced all of that and more. Everyone given chemotherapy is warned that a side effect is hair loss, but nothing can prepare a woman for the shock of baldness. She bore up under the strain with all the dignity and grace she could manage, although I know she was devastated. Little did I know that even then, my sister was teaching me.

Her partnership with George Blumenschein gave Suzy focus. Because chemotherapy and radiation are given in cycles so that a patient can have alternate periods of treatment and rest, she was able to go home and spend time with her family between trips to Houston. While at home she tried to live as normal a life as possible, with the exception of a surgery to remove a small portion of her right lung where the cancer had invaded. She continued her charity work and spent long afternoons at the hospital in Peoria sitting with terminally ill patients. To this day I hear from families of the people Suzy sat with. She even continued her modeling when she felt up to it, sporting a new look with a short wig. She had sores in her mouth from all the medication, her arm was painful and swollen from lymphedema (swelling of the arm caused by removal of the axillary lymph nodes or by radiation therapy), and she had put on weight from the steroids used to slow her cancer, but Suzy still looked beautiful. I don't think I was ever more proud of my sister.

My mother, Stan, and I tried our best to be with her while she was in Houston. If we all couldn't be there together, one of us would be there at all times. She never went alone. There was a hotel apartment across the street from the medical center where patients stayed during their courses of chemotherapy and radiation. Besides being a lot less expensive than staying every night in the hospital, it gave the patient a little bit of freedom. On nights when Suzy wasn't feeling too sick, we were able to get out to eat or catch a movie. She was able to receive her second course of chemotherapy through what is called a Gershon or subclavian catheter. For her, it was a more comfortable way of receiving the drugs. The catheter is placed in a vein just above the clavicle (or collarbone) and remains there throughout the course. A small battery-operated pump, which is carried by the patient either around the shoulder or on a belt, automatically delivers the chemo into the vein. You see, she couldn't receive the chemotherapy in the arm on the side of her surgery; there is too high a risk of infection. In the other arm, Suzy's veins had already collapsed from continuous injections.

When she wasn't in Houston I would visit her in Peoria whenever I could. I was divorced by this time, living with my son, Eric. He was just a little boy of four then and was confused as to why I was gone so much. I tried to explain that his Aunt Suzy was very sick and needed me with her. I felt better for having always told Eric the truth, but I know it was a difficult period for him. It was a difficult time for everyone who knew and loved Suzy.

The stress and tension endured by a family involved in a serious illness is unimaginable. You know you must stick together on the crucial matters, so often the tension released is by arguing about the little things. My father had a terrible time. He could not bear the sight of his precious daughter being so ill. Like many men of his generation, it was not easy for Dad to express his feelings openly. It was impossible for him to accept the fact that in this case he was not the one in control. As a result, it was our dear mother who bore much of the burden. At one point, she stayed in Houston for five and a half weeks without ever seeing the outside of the hospital. She wouldn't have it any other way. Fortunately, Mom had the strength to go it alone.

"What do we live for if not to make life less difficult for each other?"

George Eliot

It was especially difficult for her because during this time the lumps in my breasts kept reappearing. I had my left breast biopsied three different times during Suzy's ordeal. Once she had to leave Suzy's side in Houston in order to be with me in Dallas. All three of my tumors were benign (noncancerous). I hated to worry my mother, but the truth is, I was scared. Every time I felt the slightest abnormality, my heart began to race. I had learned that women whose mother or sister has had breast cancer before menopause have a slightly increased risk of developing the disease.

Whenever we felt as if we couldn't go on, that the load was just too heavy, it was Suzy's grace and humor that got us through the day. She was able to find something to smile about at every turn of the road, and her infectious, warm concern was felt throughout the hospital.

The one thing Suzy never found humor in, however, was the aesthetic conditions of the waiting rooms. The walls were empty, the chairs were uncomfortable, and sometimes a patient would have to sit there waiting for six or more hours for a scheduled appointment. Suzy was horrified and so was I. She was more concerned with the treatment of the patients; but my concern was the treatment of the disease. I was outraged that more hadn't been learned to help my sister. "Nan," she said, "as soon as I get better, let's do something about this. You can find a way to speed up the research. I know you can. And I want to fix up this waiting room and make it pretty for the women who have to be here. This isn't right."

For about fifteen months, the Houston team of Blumenschein and his associates was successful in slowing down her breast cancer. But then, for reasons known only to God, the disease started to rage inside her once again. Fully aware of her condition, but never willing to give up or talk about it, Suzy began a perilous and painful downhill battle. There was more surgery and more chemotherapy, but by now her body had built up a resistance to the drugs. Her cancer had gotten so far out of control that it broke through the skin, resulting in grotesque sores all over her chest. Her breast implant had to be replaced with some muscle from her back to restore the chest area. Plastic surgery after plastic surgery was performed to cover up these lesions. She also had an operation called an oophorectomy, which is the removal of the ovaries. In some cases an oophorectomy has been proven quite successful in slowing down the growth of the disease because certain types of breast cancer feed off female hormones. In some cases—but not Suzy's. She began to spend more time feeling awful, and we spent more time feeling helpless. None of us knew what to do anymore. Up until this point we had always spoken enthusiastically about our future together. It was becoming more obvious with each new day that this *was* our future with Suzy.

I remember one afternoon at M. D. Anderson, we were walking from the hospital over to the hotel. Suzy had just been through an awful experience. Her lungs had started to fill with fluid, and I watched as nearly a gallon of fluid was drained from them to keep her from drowning. It was very painful for her, and I could barely stand to hear her gasping for breath. The street we had to cross was quite a busy one, and as we waited for the light to change I saw a large bus barreling our way just about to pass where Suzy and I were standing. For a split second I contemplated the thought of how much easier it would be on her if she were to *accidentally fall* in front of that bus and end it all. I remembered her saying to me a long time ago that if she ever had to go through what Aunt Rose went through that she would want me to find a way to kill her. She'd rather be dead. I'm sure many of us have had similar thoughts, but when it actually happens the will to live becomes much stronger than anything else in the world. She wanted to fight, and I wanted my sister with me for as long as possible *regardless* of the circumstances. *But the reality of cancer is that it really can get that bad.*

Another afternoon during the time when Suzy stayed in Houston, we were lying together by the pool at the hotel. She loved to sunbathe as often as possible, because she felt that having color on her face was the only thing that made her look healthy. As I watched her lying there reading, I took note of her thin, frail body and strained breathing. Fortunately, Suzy was *into* her book and paid no attention to me. Had she looked over, she would have seen my tears and known immediately what I was thinking. Our time together was drawing to a close. In a flood of beautiful memories I began to look back on the wonderful relationship I shared with my sister. Frantically, I wrote my memories down, fearing somehow, I might forget one later. I didn't realize then that memories, so special, are never forgotten. I also didn't realize that what I was writing that sunny afternoon was my sister's eulogy.

In quiet desperation, my parents, Stan, and I went to Suzy's and Stan's rabbi for advice. He told us not to give up encouraging Suzy; to keep trying; but that under no circumstances were we to lie to her. It was time to begin saying our good-byes. Our family had always been totally honest with each other, and breaking that trust at this point would hurt Suzy much more than help her.

While she never gave up her fight, Suzy had to face the possibility that she might not win her war. In those last weeks, her thoughts were constantly of Stan and the children. The idea of leaving them behind was almost too much for her to bear. On one particularly bad day, she talked to Mom about Scott and Stephanie. "I worked so hard for them," she cried, "I'll never know what happened." Although Suzy may have feared this at the time, I've taken comfort in my conviction that somehow Suzy has been there all along watching over her children.

But as Suzy's illness took its toll, it was Mom who was there to put an arm around a little shoulder or hold a small hand when Suzy couldn't. She willingly accepted the impossible task of trying to mend two little broken hearts. Scott, now ten, didn't like to talk about his mother's illness. He would go off in a corner by himself and cry. Stephanie was still only six, but I think she sensed something sad and terrible was happening to her family. Thank God Mom was there for them just as she always had been for Suzy and me.

TAKING CHARGE OF BREAST CANCER

Not long after the discussion with our rabbi, I was home in Peoria visiting. One evening, my parents and Stan had taken Scott and Stephanie out to dinner, and Suzy and I were home alone. She had just come back from Houston after an intense dose of chemo. I could hear her being violently ill in the bathroom. Throughout her three-year illness, Suzy was very brave and always maintained a great deal of pride in her appearance. I knew she preferred to be left alone at times like this. But on that particular night she just kept getting sicker and sicker and pretty soon I couldn't take it anymore. I ran into the bathroom and held her in my arms. "Oh, Nan," she sobbed, "Isn't this awful? Don't I look horrible?"

"Yes, Suzy, it is horrible," I cried with her. "I don't know why this is happening to you."

After my sister was released from M. D. Anderson, I tried to come home every other week for a visit. Although she was too weak to get out of the car, Suzy insisted on riding with my parents to and from the airport when I came into town. Even though she could do little more than lie there in the back seat, this was her way of saying that she was still capable of taking care of me and that she was still there for me if I needed her.

One particular Sunday afternoon on the way back to the airport, Suzy spoke to me again about doing something to help the sick women in the hospital. This practically tore my heart out because here she was, hardly able to manage a whisper, and she was worrying about other people. I couldn't bear it. When my father pulled up to the curb, I quickly kissed them both good-bye and jumped out of the car. I was just about inside the airport when I heard a funny sound that sounded like my name. I stopped in my tracks and turned around. There was Suzy, standing up outside the car on wobbly knees, wig slightly askew. With her arms outstretched, she said gently, " Good-bye, Nanny. I love you." I hugged her so hard I was afraid she might crumble. And then I ran to catch my plane.

I never saw my sister alive again. After nine operations, three courses of chemotherapy, and radiation, she had lost her three-year war. By the time I flew back to her side it was too late. She was gone.

Mother and I went to the funeral home to say a final farewell in private before her services began. When I approached Suzy, lying there so peacefully, I was shocked when I got close enough to see her face. My shock quickly changed to fury. Whoever had applied her makeup must have been the only person in Peoria who didn't know my sister. Her face looked overly made-up and plastic, not at all like the soft, gentle woman we all loved so dearly. I insisted they remove all the makeup from her face at once. And then, alone, with my own cosmetics, I put Suzy's makeup on just the way she had taught me to do my own so many years before. Mom sat off to the side and just watched, while silent tears rolled down her cheeks.

The months after Suzy's funeral were the saddest in my life. I wanted to stay near my parents because I knew they needed me (the truth is, we needed each other), but I had a son and a home that had been without attention for too long. It was time to get on with it, to pick myself up and start living again. I owed that to Eric. Yet some things are easier said than done.

I spent a lot of time thinking about Suzy. There is no way to describe accurately the void her absence left in my life. I also spent a great deal of time questioning my faith and wondering why such a good person was taken from a family that needed her so desperately. I often wondered, as many people do when they've lost a loved one, what really happens to a soul when a person dies. Was Suzy watching me? Did she hear me when I called her name out loud? After much searching, I came to the conclusion that I would never know until I died myself, but I sure as hell didn't want to die in order to find out. Just in case, I wanted to do something to let her know how special she would always be in my heart. I was haunted by our last conversation and lay awake sometimes all night wondering what I could do to help other women with breast cancer. *Could one person really make a difference?*

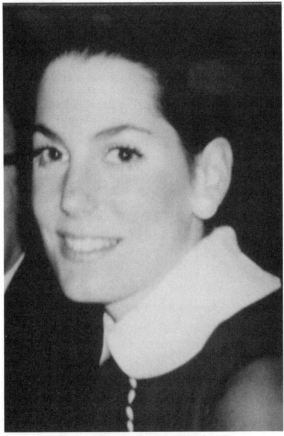

Susan G. Komen

Chapter Two
My Story

"Although the world is full of suffering it is also full of the overcoming of it."
Helen Keller

At a time when I needed a friend more than anything else in my life, in November of 1980, I met a man named Norman Brinker. Norman was and still is an extremely successful businessman in Dallas. I knew he was an eligible bachelor and had seen him at several charity functions in the city. What I had no way of knowing about was the depth of his character and the quality of his spirit.

From our first conversation, we knew we had a special bond. Norman had been married to tennis star Maureen (Little Mo) Connolly and lost her to ovarian cancer in 1969. He, more than anyone else, understood my loss. We could talk about anything and everything, and we did. Norman taught me to laugh again, something for which I will never be able to thank him adequately. What seemed like a whirlwind courtship to most of our friends seemed perfectly right to us. We had a great deal in common, including our love of horses, skiing, and politics. Norman and I married on Valentine's Day 1981.

Of course, I thought of Suzy on that happy day. I wished she could have known Norman, but somehow, I felt her beside me as I spoke my vows. The grieving

TAKING CHARGE OF BREAST CANCER

process was far from over for me, but I began to feel like myself again after Norman and I married. As happy as I was as Norman's wife, however, I found myself haunted by my promise to Suzy to do something to change the way women with breast cancer were treated in this country and make everyone more aware of its devastating toll. I didn't have the faintest idea where to begin. Norman's business acumen helped me find my way. He zeroed in on my extensive fund-raising experience for a number of different charities. "Nancy," he asked me, "Why don't you put your energy into the cause that is so dear to *your* heart?" I decided I would start a charity solely dedicated to breast cancer research. Norman was very supportive of the idea and said: "Sure, it's okay with me, but please don't call my friends." Of course, the next day when he left for work, I called every one of them. And my own contacts, too. I wasn't shy about asking for money. I just thought to myself, *I'm doing it for Suzy*. What I didn't expect was the reaction I got.

Breast cancer, at that time, was the second leading killer of women over age 44 in the United States. Yet even in 1981, ten years after the feminist movement had kicked into high gear, the subject of breast cancer was rarely raised in a public setting. I was very sure that most of my friends had no idea that over 138,000 new cases of the disease were detected every year in the U.S., or that women were facing very poor odds. In 1940, one in twenty women were diagnosed with the disease in their lifetime; but by 1981, the figure had reached one in thirteen.

Throughout my sister's three-year illness, I had learned a lot about breast cancer, but I knew that if I expected people in Dallas to reach into their pockets, I'd better know a lot more about the disease scientifically. I studied with a vengeance. I burned up the phones to the National Institutes of Health asking for information. "Send me everything!" I told them. Then I read it. All of it. For a while, I'm sure I wasn't the most popular guest at parties. I couldn't help myself. If a question started off about politics or child care, I'd somehow manage to turn it around to mammography and mastectomy—not exactly typical cocktail talk. I not only found the statistics of breast cancer horrifying, I was shocked at how little people knew or seemed to want to know about this enemy. The subject made people extremely squeamish, especially men. If it weren't such a serious matter, I would have been amused. They can talk about war with no problem. Murder is interesting. Bankruptcy is fascinating. But breast cancer? Next subject! I've always had the feeling that women's breasts are an easy topic of conversation for men among themselves or in the bedroom, but discussing them with women in an objective manner is a different story altogether.

Yes, I had my work cut out for me. It was clear that I also had to raise the awareness of women and get their support in order to get my program off the ground. It didn't take me long to realize that I couldn't do this alone. I sent out an S.O.S. to a few friends who had a similar passion for the cause because of a personal or family connection to breast cancer. They came running, and we began what became the race of our lives—a race for the cure for breast cancer that continues today. At that point, however, we weren't exactly sure what it was we were going to create. But our hearts were in the right place; and so, with two hundred dollars in cash, a borrowed typewriter, and a shoe box full of names, we launched what would become the Susan G. Komen Breast Cancer Foundation.

By the end of 1983, with a lot of hard work and a great deal of luck, we had turned that two hundred dollars into one hundred fifty thousand dollars.[1] Former First Lady

---

1. At the end of its first twenty years, we're estimating that the Foundation and its Affiliates will have raised more than 400 million dollars.

Betty Ford had graciously joined our efforts and was instrumental in helping to make the country more aware of the disease. Because of her influence over my sister and the bravery and strength she exuded throughout her own battle with breast cancer, we established the Betty Ford Award in her honor. This annual award is given by Mrs. Ford herself to a person or organization that has made significant contributions in the fight against breast cancer. Additionally, we established several scientific awards to nurture promising treatment breakthroughs throughout the country. As the reputation of the Susan G. Komen Breast Cancer Foundation grew, we began receiving requests for help from some of the most respected researchers in America. I cannot begin to explain the thrill of seeing our efforts make a difference. Twenty years have gone by since that first meeting in my living room, but we remain a volunteer-oriented organization that has become one of the nation's leaders in the fight against breast cancer. In the next chapter, I'll go into more detail about Komen's twenty years on the front lines in the battle against breast cancer.

Not long after the Komen Foundation came into being, however, I found myself fighting my own personal battle with the disease that had killed my sister. My focus had been only on fulfilling my promise to Suzy, yet my personal fear of breast cancer was never far from my mind.

One cold night in January 1984, Norman and I had just gotten into bed and I was pulling the comforter up over us in an attempt to get warm, when purely by accident and without any forewarning, as my hand skimmed lightly over my chest, I felt a small, hard lump in my left breast. I sprang out of bed, screaming, "Oh my God, I have a lump!" Norman immediately knew exactly what to do. He told me to calm down. Then, he said to call M. D. Anderson in the morning and fly to Houston to have it checked out. If it hadn't been close to midnight, I would have gone right then. At the crack of dawn the next morning, I had Fred Ames on the phone. Fred is a surgeon at M. D. Anderson whom I asked to monitor my breasts. I had already become a minor medical case study in Houston because of my family history as well as my own history of benign breast tumors. I had immense respect for Dr. Ames's work and a high regard for him personally. I told him this lump felt different from the others and that I was very concerned. He said for me to get on the next plane and come down.

After feeling my breast and reviewing my mammogram, Dr. Ames said, "Nancy, I don't think it's anything to worry about. I really feel like it's another benign tumor. I hate for you to keep having this breast biopsied because it has been done three times already, and you've got so much scar tissue now, it is going to be difficult to see what we've got in there. Let's watch it for a little while and see if it changes."

Well, I took his advice and went back to Dallas. I knew Dr. Ames had good logical, medical reasoning behind his decision. But I had become an expert in the normal changes of my own breasts, and I knew *this lump was different.* The other three had felt rubbery and this one was very hard.

Sometimes in life there are odd coincidences that simply can't be explained. Karma, fate, the hand of God at work? Who knows, but the next day, I found myself scheduled to attend a seminar on breast cancer detection sponsored by the Foundation. As you entered the room where the seminar was to take place, there were display tables set up with all kinds of written material for the guests to take with them. There were also several breast forms with hidden lumps in them so that the women could come by and feel exactly what we were talking about. As I stood there welcoming our guests, my hand fell behind me absently, and I unconsciously began to feel the forms. Surprisingly enough, I had never done this before. I came across something that felt a little too familiar. One of the lumps in the form felt very much like the one in my own breast. Panic nearly caused me to run for the exit. But somehow I managed to hold on and stay focused that day. Ironically, I was speaking to a group of women on how important it is to be vigilant about our breast health. I wondered what they would say if they knew that, at that very moment, I thought I had a serious problem.

After the seminar, I went to see my surgeon in Dallas, Morris Fogelman. Dr. Fogelman had removed my previous three lumps and really knew my history. He was aware of the fact that I had since become a case study at M. D. Anderson, but I had always been very comfortable with him and just wanted another opinion. He said, "Nancy, that does not feel good to me, and if I were you, I'd get it out." I didn't want to overact, and I had to take into consideration that Dr. Fogelman had said the same thing about my other three lumps, but I had a feeling he was right. He took me upstairs and did a test called transillumination (also known as diaphonography), which involves shining a bright light through the breast to illuminate its interior. Different types of tissues transmit and scatter the light in different ways. The test is read on an infrared-sensitive television camera. Studies indicate that transillumination, however, is unable to detect the tinier lumps regularly found in mammography. I felt the test was unnecessary for me.

I already knew I had a lump and wasn't looking for confirmation. What I wanted to know was whether or not I had cancer. Unfortunately, that could only be determined at that point by a needle biopsy. Still, the radiologist who read the test said he, too, felt that my tumor was benign because it was a very round lump with clear definition all the way around it. The name *cancer* is derived from a Latin word meaning *crab*. When you picture a crab in your mind, its claws and legs reach out away from its body. The disease cancer is thought to do the same thing. It often spreads out in all directions, invading the healthy tissues and organs of the body. That is why having a perfectly round, clearly defined lump can be a good sign.

Once again, I went home and tried to act normally as I waited for the results. I don't think I went fifteen minutes all day without poking or feeling that lump. I swore to myself I could feel it growing. Ten days later I went back to Dr. Fogelman. He said, "Nancy, it *is* getting bigger; get it out of there." Immediately, I called Fred Ames and told him I wanted this thing out—no matter what it was. He said, "No problem. Come on down—we'll do it here in the office. I feel very confident about its being benign, but I know you're troubled, so let's get rid of it. I'll give you a local anesthetic and do a biopsy right here in my office."

Norman was in Florida on business, and my parents were also there where they spend most of the winter. I called and told them I was going to Houston, but that Dr. Ames felt sure there was nothing to be concerned over. Convincing them that I wasn't worried was truly an Oscar®-winning performance. The truth was that I had a very uneasy feeling in the pit of my stomach. No, the real truth was that I was petrified. The same instincts of mine that had raised flags when Suzy was diagnosed were kicking in again, this time for me.

I was greeted at M. D. Anderson by Doris Bechtold, one of the patient-care coordinators at the hospital, a woman who had treated me and my family as her own from the first day we brought Suzy in the door. Dr. Ames brought me right into the day surgery room. I was given a local anesthetic so that I was completely awake and alert. A short curtain was placed directly under my chin. I couldn't see the actual surgery, but I stared into Fred Ames's eyes for the entire operation, searching for a clue. I decided he must be a world-class poker player; he didn't give me so much as a raised eyebrow. When a biopsy is done the suspicious tissue is mounted and sent to the pathology department for analysis. Some of the tissue is frozen and mounted on a slide for an immediate microscopic examination. Through the examination of the "frozen section," results may be determined in a matter of minutes. Analyzing the "permanent section" of the tissue can take several days. I wanted my results as quickly as possible, so I asked for both. I was wheeled into the recovery room where I waited for what seemed like forever, but was probably less than an hour. All of a sudden, Dr. Ames came through the door as I sat there with a brave smile on my face that I didn't feel. I'm sure every one of my fingers was crossed as I looked up at him and said, "Another false alarm, right?" It seemed as if time had stopped, and it was someone else sitting there waiting to hear if she would live or die.

He took a deep breath and said, " No, Nancy, it's not good news. It's cancer."

Suddenly, everything was real again. I remember leaping off the bed and screaming, "Tell me you're not telling me this! Tell me you're kidding! Please tell me what you're saying is not the truth!" And then I sobbed. My head was pounding as I was overwhelmed by memories of Suzy and my own fears.

He walked over, hugged me, and said quietly, "Nancy, I sent it back twice because I didn't want to believe the diagnosis, but it is confirmed. You've got cancer. Now, I want you to calm down. It was very small, and I think we've gotten it very early. You have a lot of options."

I just remember screaming, "I want them both off today. Get them off me! I want them off now!" I was so scared and so angry and so upset.

Calmly, Fred told me to get dressed, call Norman and my mother, and then we could talk about the situation rationally. I couldn't reach Norman, but I did reach my mother. She said that she would get Norman, and they would both be there on the next flight. All I could think of was Suzy. I remembered how she didn't want a mastectomy and how desperately afraid I was of following in her footsteps.

Mom asked me what I wanted to do, and I told her, "Get rid of both breasts." Then I talked with Fred, and he said he really didn't feel that was necessary. I was aware, even then, of a procedure called "lumpectomy," which was finally receiving the appropriate amount of attention and study it deserved through many years of exhaustive work by a physician named Bernard Fisher. A lumpectomy is a surgical procedure in which only the cancerous tumor and a small amount of the surrounding tissue is removed. It is usually followed by radiation and sometimes other forms of *adjuvant therapy* (treatment other than surgery). When a lumpectomy is a clinical option, it may save a woman from losing her breast. Unfortunately, the cosmetic advantages of a lumpectomy, in my case, did not apply. I knew that if I could get through this alive, down the road I would have reconstructive surgery. To be honest, how I would end up looking was not a priority at the time. I simply didn't want to die.

I checked myself into the hospital right away and went through a whole battery of other tests. They did a full body X ray, a bone scan, and another chest X ray to see if the cancer had metastasized to other areas of my body. Doris Bechtold and Fred Ames never left my side. All the tests came out negative, but I couldn't allow myself to relax because I knew my lymph nodes hadn't been tested yet and wouldn't be until the surgery the next day. George Blumenschein was away on a ski vacation.

By the time my mother and Norman arrived that evening, I was sedated, wailing, frightened, and confused. Both of them looked me in the eye and said they *knew* I'd be all right. Mom says now that she really did have a different feeling about my outcome. She never admitted her true fear during Suzy's illness, but it was always there. Unlike Suzy, when I was diagnosed, she believed deep down, I would survive. I wanted to believe it, and I found myself already imagining myself well again. Still, I couldn't afford to be too optimistic. Breast cancer is serious business. The mental picture of Suzy at the end of her life, so small, shriveled, and weak, was haunting me. I was ready to fight, and I wanted to get on with it. But that night I just wanted to be cuddled because the next day I was declaring war.

Mother spent the night with me in the hospital. My breast burned from the biopsy, but I kept touching it anyway, thinking it would be the last time I'd be able to feel any sensation at all on that side of my chest. Remembering Scott and Stephanie's reaction, I worried about Eric knowing how frightened and alone he must feel. I thought about Norman and knew, although he'd never say, how frightened *he* must be after already having lived through the loss of one wife with cancer. And then I looked over at my mother, so brave and cheerful in the next bed. What must she be thinking? Was she preparing herself psychologically to lose another daughter after a long and gruesome illness? The answer was no! When she looked at me and said I would be fine, I searched her eyes for signs of untruth or pity. There were none.

The next thing I remember is being wheeled into the operating room the following morning. I touched my breast one more time before going under, and then it was over. When I was wheeled back to my room, it was filled with people and flowers. I went to sleep feeling loved, calm, and content to be alive.

It must have been the anesthesia because that contented feeling didn't last. The next morning I woke up wanting to get going, to do whatever it was that had to be done in order to get well. Dr. Ames came to see me and said that although my nodes looked clear to him, the official results wouldn't be back for a couple of days. He also told me that he had made the incision in a place where reconstruction would be easy should I decide to have it done down the road. I couldn't see anything at that point because my entire chest was bandaged down to my waist. With all those bandages I couldn't even tell that one of my breasts was missing. What I felt was a hot, burning sensation all over my chest. There were tubes protruding from the wrapping on my left side to allow the excess fluid to be drained from my body. It is the body's natural response to automatically send fluid to a vacant pocket of flesh. At first there is too much fluid to be reabsorbed naturally, so the tubes are usually left in place for three or four days.

I wasn't in pain; I guess this is where the term *uncomfortable* comes into play. Mostly I was restless. I wanted to do something. My family and friends were babying me, treating me like a sick person—and I didn't feel sick. The first moment I was alone, I got out of bed and took a walk through the hospital and upstairs to the physical therapy room. I knew exactly where it was because I had been there with Suzy. I got on a stationary bike and was able to pedal a couple of miles before one of my nurses found me and demanded I get back in bed. There was a precious little boy in the room who couldn't have been more than three years old. My heart ached for this small boy. I looked at his lost little face and thought how unfair it was that he couldn't be outdoors playing with other boys. I thought about how Suzy would have reacted if she had seen him. It would have broken her heart.

So would the looks on the faces of the other recovering patients doing their daily exercises. I hadn't seen that many bored looks since some of my first cold calls trying to raise money for the Foundation. As I stood there, I could almost hear Suzy's voice whispering in my ear again: "Do something, Nan." The next day, I bought six portable tape players and headsets for the therapy room— another installment on my promise to Suzy. I figured if music is good for the soul, why not the body, too?

Anyone who has had cancer or knows anyone who has had cancer or even has read anything about people with cancer will hear one thing over and over again: This is a disease that makes a person feel completely out of control. When you get a cold or the flu you can usually feel it coming on. You know the probable outcome, and you can prepare for it, if not avoid it. But cancer is something you can't prepare for. By the time you know you've got it, the disease has quietly invaded your body without warning. I call it the stealth disease. There are things I did in an effort to take control of my body, which I am sure other people would not choose to do.

"When the heart grieves over what it has lost, the spirit rejoices in what it has left."

Sufi Epigram

Remember, I was a very well-educated cancer patient at the time, and I had seen the disease at its worst. But nothing could have prepared me for the shock and fear of discovering breast cancer in my own body. I thought I understood it because I was so close to Suzy, but in truth, I didn't. Each case is special. It comes with its own set of specifics, both medical and emotional. All I was certain of was that I would do *anything* I could to rid myself of this breast cancer and get on with my life.

George Blumenschein was at my side within a couple of days following my surgery. He had spoken to Fred Ames, seen my lab reports, and, as is typically Blumenschein, gave it to me straight—chapter and verse. He said: "Nancy, I think you are in a good situation. There was no node involvement and your tumor was still small. I feel very optimistic about your case, but I am going to recommend we treat this very aggressively for a number of reasons. First of all, your age. As a rule, the younger the patient, the more aggressive the cancer. Thirty-six is young to have breast cancer. And while your tumor was not wildly aggressive, it showed signs of being on the aggressive side, which can mean rapid growth. We also have to take into consideration the fact that your hormone receptor assay was negative [a hormone receptor assay is a test done at the time of the biopsy to determine whether or not a breast cancer's growth is influenced by female hormones], and your previous family history with the disease is very important. I want to bring you from an 85 percent survival rate to a 95 percent survival rate. And for that I recommend four courses of chemotherapy, to begin as soon as possible after your surgery heals."

He went on to explain that if I agreed to this form of treatment, I would lose all my hair and possibly experience other unpleasant side effects. Some people develop leukemia from chemotherapy; sometimes the hair may not grow back all the way. Some people get violently sick from the drugs, while others make it through the treatments with a minimal amount of discomfort.

Dr. Blumenschein assigned me to a protocol—a combination of drugs given at a set time in set dosages—being used in a clinical trial he was conducting at M. D. Anderson. I would be given several forms of chemotherapy including Adriamycin, 5-Flurouracil (also known as 5-FU), and Cytoxan. In chapter 8, I will explain more about these and other forms of chemotherapy, but for now what is important to know is that the protocol called for high dosages of strong drugs intended to kill off fast-growing cells aggressively. Dr. Blumenschein also explained to me that since Suzy's illness, improvements had been made in the subclavian catheter and pump. He said I could be very mobile if I chose this method of drug delivery and that there was a class available at M. D. Anderson where I could learn everything I needed to know about administering the drugs myself in the safest way possible. I did take the class, and I did have the catheter surgically implanted. It's amazing what you find yourself capable of when your very life is at stake. I wanted to go home to Eric and Norman and give them back the mother and wife they had counted on. At the time, nothing else mattered.

I am a lucky woman. I had the means to get the best medical treatment available. And I was educated enough to know how to find it. Still, there were those who didn't agree with the treatment I chose. Some highly respected members of the medical community thought perhaps my treatment was *too* aggressive. Maybe I didn't need a modified radical mastectomy; a lumpectomy may have been equally effective. Perhaps I didn't need such a strong dosage of chemotherapy. What the outcome would have been with a less aggressive treatment, I will never know, but to those who think I should have handled it differently, all I can say is, "I'm still here" and I'm not one to second-guess success.

I made an informed decision that was mine to make. I was fully aware of all my options. Between Fred Ames and George Blumenschein, I had a highly qualified medical team I believed in. I trusted their advice, but that's what it was—advice. I had to do what I felt was right for me. It was funny because when Suzy was so sick, I looked at her and thought to myself, *I could never go through this. I could never voluntarily submit my body to such torture.* But when push came to shove and I was faced with the same life-threatening disease, the choices were not difficult. Besides having medical options and much more education, I was lucky in other ways which proved to be equally as important. I had good friends and a lot of people depending on me to get better. I had built the Susan G. Komen Breast Cancer Foundation not only in the hope of one day finding a cure, but with the intention of helping women make informed decisions about their own breast health. I not only wanted to fight this disease, I wanted to beat this disease with every fiber of my being. My reputation depended on it. This is not to say that I recommend my form of treatment to anyone else. Each woman has to decide for herself which options best serve her needs. She has to assemble her own team of medical experts and make her informed decision based on their advice.

My team consisted of more than medical experts. I had a strong support team of emotional and spiritual members as well. I don't know what I would have done without my mother's help. She was with me every step of the way, and still is to this day. Norman convinced me that he would love me exactly the same with or without both breasts. I had friends who kept me laughing throughout the whole ordeal, which could have been, perhaps, the best medicine of all. One afternoon shortly after my surgery, I found myself alone in the room quietly contemplating my future. The phone next to my bed rang, and it was Betty Ford. She wanted to know how I was doing. Immediately, I began to fight back the tears. The more she spoke, the more emotional I became. I was embarrassed and told her so. I will never forget her words. She said: "Nancy, allow yourself the luxury of tears. Cry your heart out and say all those things you're feeling. Really pity yourself and ask, 'Why me?' You need to do all of that . . . but only for one day. Get it all out of your system and then release it. Let it go. You have studied this disease like no one else. You know what you have to do. Trust yourself and believe in your good judgment. Try to get through one day at a time. If one day seems too overwhelming, try to get through it one hour at a time. The rest is up to God, whatever 'God' means to you. There is a line from the twenty-third Psalm that goes, 'Though I walk through the valley of the shadow of death . . .' Nancy, it says you walk through it, it doesn't say you have to stop there. You have a whole lot of people who love you very much and are pulling for you to recover."

When I hung up the phone, I took Mrs. Ford's advice and cried my heart out. I cried for Suzy and for Eric and for my parents and for Norman. I cried for myself. The next day I checked out of the hospital.

It was time to start taking control. I didn't go straight home. My mother and I went wig shopping. Around Dallas, the word had spread like wildfire that I had cancer. I was already being called for radio and television interviews to discuss my disease and how I was planning to handle it. I thought the better I looked, the more positive the message I would send out. My first stop was the hairdresser's where I told him, "Cut it off." I think he thought I'd lost my mind, or I was still on drugs. The fact was that the wigs I had purchased were short styles, and I wanted the transition to look as smooth as possible.

This is something I had to do for me. It wasn't as if no one knew my hair was going to fall out. Of course, everyone I was close to knew what was happening. It was more a matter of preserving my dignity. I didn't want to give people any more reason to pity me. Letting myself go would have been, in my eyes, surrendering to the disease. I was determined to stay one step—no, several steps—ahead of my cancer.

It was also very important to look good for Eric. Poor little Eric was so frightened. All he knew was that his Aunt Suzy had had breast cancer, and she died. Now his mother had the same disease. He didn't understand the fact that mine was detected and treated much earlier than Suzy's or that my tumor was much smaller and not nearly as aggressive. At eight years old, none of that mattered to him. I believed that the best thing I could do for him was to convince him that I felt well.

My mother volunteered to come back to M. D. Anderson with me for the four courses of chemotherapy. I felt awful putting her through the same hell she knew all too well, but she insisted. To be honest, I couldn't think of anyone else I'd rather have with me.

Like Suzy, I was confined to the hospital. For the first part of the treatment I received a combination of 5-FU and Cyoxan delivered through an IV drip directly into the subclavian catheter. That was followed by four days of continuous infusion of Adriamycin through a small pump. I was given four vials of the drug to take with me over to the hospital hotel. As each of the vials emptied onto the catheter a little signal went off to let me know it was time to make the change. It was kind of a tricky procedure because the catheter has to be meticulously cleaned in order to prevent infection. I am not mechanically inclined at all and didn't enjoy fiddling with it. Mother was very helpful and made sure the job was done right. That night I felt pretty good, so Mom and I went out for dinner. I was in the mood for a juicy hamburger and fries, a treat I don't often allow myself. But I felt I deserved it, so we threw our diets to the wind and indulged. By the time we got to bed, I was content and tired, looking forward to a good night's sleep. It wasn't to be. At three o'clock in the morning I woke up violently ill, with the most wretched, flu-like symptoms you could imagine. I was ill over and over again until I began to dehydrate, and Mother took me right back to the clinic. They gave me an IV and soda with chipped ice, and they put me on an anti-nausea drug.

Suzy used to complain of having a metallic taste in her mouth after chemotherapy and now I knew what she meant. I became acutely sensitive to all kinds of smells— things that never bothered me before could make me turn absolutely green. It was a pretty ghastly experience, but before long I had finished my first round and was home again in Dallas. They sent me home with all kinds of antidepressants, Valium and who knows what else, to try to relieve some of the side effects of the chemo. I tried to take as little medicine as possible. I've never been one to take a lot of pills, and I wanted to save the drugs for times when I really needed them because I know your body can build up an immunity toward certain medications. For the first few days, I felt mildly flu-like, and then I started to feel good again. I got dressed every day, and although I wasn't up for aerobics, I made it a personal goal at least to get out and walk, even if it was just for a short time.

Nine days after my first round of chemotherapy, I was sitting in front of the mirror brushing my hair when it happened. I looked at the brush, and it was filled with

my little short hairs. Intellectually, I knew the loss of my
hair was only a matter of time, but I didn't fully understand the emotional shock until I experienced it myself.
A huge wave of panic overtook my whole body. It didn't
matter that I knew it was coming or that I was prepared
for it. The truth is, I don't think you can ever be *really*
prepared for going bald. That first day I was probably the
only one who noticed any difference at all. I was terrified
of what Eric would think. I didn't want him to be afraid
of me. The next day, it was even worse—lots more hair in
the brush. I felt completely out of control and that the
disease was gaining on me. I was there alone in my room
crying, feeling terribly sorry for myself. Then I remembered Mrs. Ford's encouraging words. It was time to
take control and get on with my life. I stood up, got into
a steaming hot shower, and finished the job myself. I
yanked every hair out of my head before it could fall out
on its own. Then I sat in front of the mirror again and
stared at my head from all angles until I was comfortable
with the new me, or at least as comfortable as I would
ever get. I wanted to deal with the situation and face the
facts. *As a side effect to getting rid of my breast cancer, I was
going to be temporarily bald. I could handle it!*

I did my best to keep my round, bald head covered up
at all times. I wore scarves and turbans, and my wigs. As
time went on, I became more relaxed about the hair
thing, though I never went to bed bareheaded. Besides
the obvious reason of wanting to look as appealing as
possible to Norman, it should be duly noted that a bald
head is a cold head. You have no idea unless you've been
through it how cold your body can get without hair. And
just for the record, your head isn't the only place you
lose it. I felt I looked more like a plucked chicken than a
woman. Eric did walk in my bedroom once and see my
head before I could get covered up, and I know he was

really jolted. But that soon passed and before too long, he was back to acting like an eight-year-old boy. Sometimes when I was getting ready to leave the house, Eric would come over innocently to kiss me good-bye, and yank off my wig and run off with it. Naturally, I'd run after him screaming and soon we'd end up on the floor laughing until the tears streamed from our eyes. I was enormously grateful for those silly times because it proved that our relationship transcended the disease. I know I often took the anger I was feeling about being burdened with breast cancer out on Eric and Norman. Sometimes in our frustration at having to fight every minute of every day, we forget our families are hurting, too. And while sharing it might have been a normal reaction, it wasn't fair to them.

Once I had adjusted to my new "look," I found myself wanting to return to my old life as soon as possible. Although I had months of chemotherapy ahead of me, I longed for the challenge of my work. As soon as I got a green light from my physicians, I went back to the Komen Foundation and resumed as many responsibilities as possible. In my mind, I had to prove that I was the ideal cancer patient and that meant getting myself back into saddle and taking charge of my life once again.

When April came, it was time for me to go back to Houston for Round Two. I had come up with another idea I was anxious to discuss with George Blumenschein. As much as I know the automatic pump is a remarkable device for many patients and most people love it, I really didn't feel it was the best option for me. I realize the pump allows patients their freedom to continue with more or less as normal a life as possible, but I am an impatient woman and wanted the whole thing over with yesterday. More importantly, I didn't like the idea of giving myself the medication. Quite frankly, I didn't trust myself to do it right, and I was tired of burdening my mother with the responsibility. What I wanted to do was check myself into M. D. Anderson and have Dr. Blumenschein put me to sleep, speed up the process of delivery of the chemotherapy to two days, and be done with it. One night in the hospital, two days of treatment, and that's it. We discussed this idea at great length. That's one of the things I loved and still do about George Blumenschein—he always treated me with great respect and considered my opinions. We were truly partners in my treatment. He had come to know my impatience as well as anyone and understood my reasons for wanting my medication in this manner. He explained that I couldn't be knocked out completely during chemotherapy because if I got sick from the medication I could easily choke, and also that the process could only be sped up so much. So we compromised. First, I turned in the pump I used for the initial course. I was allowed to be sedated but not asleep during the treatment. I did have four days' worth of chemo administered in two days' time through an IV drip. The catheter remained in my body for the IV, but I no longer had to fiddle with it except to keep the area clean and infection free. The first time we tried this, it didn't go as smoothly as I had hoped. I still got pretty sick, but at least it was over a lot sooner. Today, thanks to new anti-nausea drugs, nausea can be controlled to a much larger degree.

There is something about recovering at home that I found particularly comforting. Looking out of my own window at my own lawn gave me a feeling of inner peace. As I enjoyed the luxuries of home and family, my mind kept bringing me back to all the other women I had seen at M. D. Anderson who were not as financially fortunate as I. Breast cancer, like all deadly diseases, is expensive. What could the Foundation do for these women? It was then, in the spring of 1984, that the idea of a low-cost screening center was born. This idea turned into reality in 1986 at Parkland Hospital in Dallas. The Komen Foundation made a $500,000, five-year grant to the hospital to open a screening clinic aimed at knocking down the barriers of accessibility and cost that often keep low-income women from getting the mammograms they need. The center provided a full range of services from diagnosis through the post-op treatment phase.

I did notice something unusual happening after my second course of chemotherapy. I was having awful "black dreams." I have since learned they are a common side effect, but I found them horrifying. I could never remember exactly what went on in the dreams but they were dark, mysterious, and ugly. I would wake in the night absolutely terrified. In order to go back to sleep I would wander into the kitchen and pour myself a glass of wine, or two. It was the first and only time I ever thought I was drinking too much. It wasn't that I was drinking huge quantities of alcohol, but two glasses of wine every day on top of the pills and chemotherapy was taking its toll on my body. We now know that a person undergoing chemotherapy should stay away from alcohol altogether. It is not good for the system to mix cytotoxic drugs and alcohol. I felt lethargic and overweight and irritable. The realization scared me to death. I cut out the wine for a long time and focused on a healthy diet and regular exercise routine. I began to feel better and noticed I was regaining my strength much faster. Much to my parents' displeasure, I even started to ride horses again. I began to set small, achievable physical goals for myself, gearing up to one big goal, which was to play in a polo match by the end of July. Norman was worried, too, but knew by now that once I had made up my mind he couldn't stop me. So he watched, and being a superb polo player himself, coached my riding and made sure I wasn't taking on too much too fast

My third and fourth courses of chemotherapy went like clockwork. After a few minor adjustments in the combinations of the medicine, Dr. Blumenschein and I had found a way to make it work. It was, for me, a great accomplishment. The euphoria of completing chemotherapy was tempered, however, by a feeling of panic that I was no longer doing anything to fight the cancer. I was, of course, thrilled to be done with the treatment, but now what was I supposed to do? Sit back and do nothing? I couldn't help remembering when Suzy thought *she* was cured. Would that happen to me? It is a bevy of mixed emotions experienced by many cancer patients. The feeling is frightening almost like the first day of school. You feel alone, timid, afraid to get back to the mainstream. I had been well taken care of by George Blumenschein, my family, and my friends. Now it was time to fly solo again, and I was scared.

"When you get to the end of your rope, tie a knot and hang on. And swing!"
Leo Buscaglia

The only thing that kept me sane was following the advice of another friend and cancer expert, the late Rose Kushner. She told me, "Nancy, always keep a full calendar. Don't give yourself a chance to worry and don't ever plan for a time when you might not be around to fulfill all the obligations you have made."

These were wise words, ones that I have repeated often to other cancer patients. This advice, in addition to striving for a physical goal, kept me going through what was an extremely difficult time. My own physical goal, which would certainly not be most people's first choice, was to play in a polo match. It was now time to prove to my friends that I was back. I threw myself into fundraising for the Komen Foundation and started to ride every day even swinging the polo mallet once again. The truth is, it felt great. Yes, I wore out easily, but I also felt invigorated and alive. When it came time to play in that match, I was ready. I'm sure I was quite a sight. There I was, bald as a billiard ball, charging down the field with nothing under my helmet but a scarf. My mother and father were standing on the side of the field with a small oxygen tank, in case of an emergency. It was a blazing hot July day in Dallas, and I guess they were afraid I would pass out from the heat. Norman and Eric were also there, watching on the sidelines. Our team won the match, and afterward, when the photographs were taken, I was the only player who didn't remove her helmet—a gesture I am sure was greatly appreciated by all. The victory, for me, had little to do with polo.

For the next year and a half, I went through what my mother terms "the checkup crazies." My friend Carolyn Walker, also a former cancer patient, calls it "toe cancer." What it means is that every tiny ache or pain is immediately assumed to be the worst. You are torn between wanting to rush to the doctor every other minute and, at the same time, being scared to death to step into his office. Dr. Blumenschein had gone into private practice in Arlington, a city right outside of Dallas. I am sure I drove him nearly out of his mind, but he was always concerned, always ready and eager to see me.

It wasn't until almost two years after my initial surgery that I really started to look at myself and think about reconstruction. After a lot of investigation, I went to a physician by the name of John Bostwick in Atlanta, Georgia. Dr. Bostwick has published several textbooks on the subject of reconstruction, and he showed me dozens of pictures of his work. His book, *A Woman's Decision*, explained in complete detail the latest reconstruction procedures. He told me how he thought the surgery should be done and how it would look. He also told me about the risks and everything that could possibly go wrong. I liked him and respected him right away.

I was extremely pleased with the results; and on the day I went to the department store to purchase my first real bra in two years, I felt as giddy as a twelve-year-old on her first trip to the lingerie department. It was fun to wear clothes that showed cleavage; I had almost forgotten what it was like. There are several types of reconstruction available now (see chapter 9), and they should be reviewed with your physician to determine what is right for you.

The one problem I had not anticipated was lymphedema, which is swelling and collection of fluid in the arm on the side of the surgery. I knew all about it, of course, and had gone to great lengths to prevent it from happening to me. I exercised my affected arm regularly, and kept it free of jewelry. I was very careful and, therefore, not the lymphedema prototype. But about a year after my reconstruction, I accidentally burned my arm on the stove. It became infected and the infection caused my arm to blow up like a balloon. It was grotesque. I don't remember ever being so mad. Here I had suffered through the cancer, endured chemotherapy, worn a prosthesis for two years, and finally had successful reconstructive surgery. I had done everything possible to look normal again, and now this.

Dr. George Peters, a Dallas breast surgeon, recommended a physical therapist, whom I saw every day. Some people told me that once an infection set in, the condition would be irreversible. George Blumenschein, too, had doubts about my recovery from lymphedema. But I wasn't going to accept it, not even from Blumenschein. As far as I was concerned, not making a complete recovery wasn't an option for me. I became even more emphatic about my diet, I exercised like a crazy person, wore an elastic sleeve on my arm all the time to try to bring the swelling down, and took antibiotics every day. Eventually, it worked, but the whole process took over a year. I am not sure that women are warned about lymphedema with enough urgency. It is a serious problem that, I feel, can disfigure a woman far more visibly than a mastectomy. To me, the surgery was easy to hide; but when one of your arms, from the shoulder to the wrist, is three times the size of your other arm, now *that's* difficult to cover up. And the *last* thing a woman needs to hear is that it is an irreversible condition. I didn't accept that, and I don't think any woman should.

Sometimes patients can teach their physicians a thing or two about medicine. George Blumenschein often talks about what I taught him on the subject of lymphedema. There have been improvements in the treatment of lymphedema since that time. Ask your physician, or a trained physical therapist about the latest treatments or combinations of treatments, and read more about it in chapter 10.

Although many have said it, it doesn't make the statement any less true; when you are told you have cancer, your life changes forever. *Forever.* I have always been a doer, always wanted to get things done yesterday. The long-term effect of having breast cancer for me has been to make me do everything in my life even faster.

I think it drives my family and friends crazy. They all tell me I don't relax enough, that I push too hard. But I can't help it. There are a lot of things I want to get done while I'm healthy enough to do them. Subconsciously, perhaps I feel that if I slow down even for a short while, I am saying to those cancer cells, "Come and get me." Still, it doesn't do you any good to worry constantly about what *might* happen. That takes all the fun out of life. I have done everything I know possible to be healthy.

In 1992, our family faced tragedy again when Norman, an athletic, active 61-year-old, nearly died from a fall during a championship polo match in Palm Beach. Norman and another rider were both galloping at top speed when the collision occurred—two half-ton horses plowing into one another on a muddy field. Norman got the short end of the deal as his smaller horse went down on its side, falling on top of him—the worst kind of polo accident. I watched in horror from the sidelines as it happened. His head hit the ground with a terrible force, and he was immediately knocked out. Norman had a habit of signaling me that he was all right after a run-in on the field. I waited to see him jump up and give me a sign with his big smile. He never moved.

I raced onto the field. The medics were just arriving. I called for oxygen, and the medics told me they didn't know how to activate it. After years of hospitals, that was something I could do and did fast. We loaded Norman into a van and rushed to the nearest emergency room. Once he was stabilized, he was flown to another hospital where he remained in a deep and life-threatening coma. His brain injuries were extensive, and at first, we thought we might actually lose him. The physicians weren't optimistic about his chances. It was touch and go for two weeks as he lay in the coma. I couldn't leave his side, and poor Eric, who loved Norman as his father, was devastated; but thankfully, Norman stuck with us. Ahead of him were months of painful and difficult physical therapy to tackle the paralysis that immobilized the left side of his body. The accident left his mind confused, and it would need a good workout, too. Norman is much too brilliant a man to do otherwise.

But as I did with my own illness, I was determined to help Norman recover completely. He had been the "wind beneath my wings" so many times, now it was my turn to be there for him. It was a terrible ordeal for Norman, for Eric and me.

Watching this vibrant man struggle with simple tasks, sitting up, standing, taking that first step was difficult. I wished I could do it for him. But I knew from my own recovery that empathy is better medicine than sympathy, and I simply would not let Norman accept anything less than a total recovery. We would do it together.

It took many months, but Norman's own determination and courage got him through his ordeal and back on his feet. Unfortunately, that's not the end of the story. He was nearly himself again when one fall morning, he decided to hop on his bike for a quick turn around the block. The worst happened. He fell and seriously reinjured himself. It meant almost starting over. I have to admit I wanted to wring his neck, but we did start over. While he never got back on a horse, Norman today is up and walking, talking like he'd never been injured, and enjoying a full life.

For me, life has always been an adventure, and as the Komen Foundation turns twenty, the adventure continues. I have been cancer-free for seventeen years, and I thank God and my physicians every single day. Eric is grown now, a wonderful young man out on his own but still the joy of my life. Sadly, Norman and I have divorced, but we remain extremely close friends. He is one of the most remarkable men I've ever known, and I will always be grateful to him for believing in me and my ability to make the Komen Foundation a reality.

> *"Life itself is the proper binge."*
>
> Julia Child,
> breast cancer survivor

Mom remains the consummate volunteer and, much to the frustration of her friends, she still refuses to play bridge, preferring to travel for Komen instead, and keeping us all going with her endless enthusiasm and common sense. Dad, at eighty-four, won't slow down either, going to his office and amazing everyone with his energy and spirit.

Suzy's husband Stan never remarried, choosing instead to focus his life on being a wonderful father. Their son Scott is a businessman in St. Louis today, is married, and is delighted to be Maddie's dad. Stephanie just signed on as a lobbyist for health care issues in Washington and spends much of her time as a dedicated Komen "angel." Both are doing fine and together were instrumental in starting the Komen Race for the Cure® in St. Louis.

And me? As I write this, I am awaiting confirmation as our country's new ambassador to Hungary. It is a great honor to have been appointed by President Bush, and I must admit I'm excited at the prospect of facing a whole new set of challenging issues in an exciting and interesting environment. But the Komen Foundation will always be the home I return to.

I have no idea what tomorrow will bring, and I don't want to wait for my future to run its course; I make it happen. If I have learned anything in my twenty years as a patient advocate, it is that life is too precious to waste a single moment.

Now you know the whole story. I said I would tell you everything, and I have. At times throughout the years, it has seemed to me and the members of my family as if we were acting out parts in some unfathomable novel rather than participating in real life. Other times we have felt so much a part of *real life* that the energy surges through our bones like a bolt of lightning. There is more to this, however, than the trauma experienced by my family. The good news is all the wonderful progress that has happened *because* of what we went through. Over the past twenty years, the thousands of women and men who make up the Susan G. Komen Breast Cancer Foundation have made enormous strides in bringing public awareness of breast cancer to the forefront. Every day we do our best to reach new women and men, and enlist more fighters in this war.

When Suzy died, she left a void in my life that still remains, but I am with her every day through the Susan G. Komen Breast Cancer Foundation. The gift she gave to me in life is one that I will cherish always, but the gift she gave in death is the one for which I will be eternally grateful. It is also the gift she gives the world. If Suzy hadn't died of breast cancer, the Komen Foundation might never have been born. It would not have become the nation's leading catalyst in the war on breast cancer, and I would not have been inspired to learn the facts that saved my life or carry out her wish to educate other women.

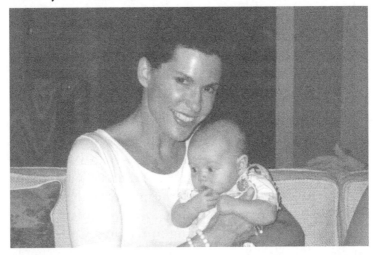

Nancy Brinker holds her great-niece, Susan Madeline Komen. Born March 14, 2000, to parents Scott and Marnie Komen, Maddie is Suzy Komen's first grandchild.

Chapter Three
The Susan G. Komen Breast Cancer Foundation's Mission

*"Never doubt that a small group of thoughtful,
committed citizens can change the world.
Indeed, it is the only thing that ever has."*
Margaret Mead

"Nothing was ever accomplished by sitting around on your duff!"

That was Ellie Goodman talking to a pair of little girls living in Peoria in the fifties; and when our mother was dispensing advice, believe me, Suzy and I listened. I still do. She taught us so many things. How to think for ourselves *and* bake cookies. How to be well-mannered young ladies *and* women ready to live life to the fullest. She and Dad gave us strong moral values that put us on the right track and gave us strength during the dark times that would come. But she also believed that what fulfills us as humans is our ability to lighten the burden for others; to make a difference in someone else's life. So, with her *own* life, by her own example, she taught us to be good stewards, to take responsibility—for ourselves, each other and for the world around us.

"You girls have to be stewards for your country," she'd tell Suzy and me. Stewards? Take care of my country? *But I'm only six*, I used to think to myself. There was

no point in arguing that kind of logic with Ellie Goodman.
Doing right by your country was a requirement at any age.

Volunteering for good causes was as much a part of
my mother's nature as was her loving concern for her
husband and children. She made time for both, and we
understood that when she was out on one of her "mis-
sions," well, that was part of our being good stewards,
too—sharing her with others.

In our family, stewardship was practically hereditary.
Mom was an only child, and her own mother was the
caretaker of the family all her life. When Mom was small,
there were few charitable organizations, and she remembers her mother often packing a basket of food or a box
of clothes to take to someone in need.

Her mother used to say, "If you have to ask what to
do, get out of the kitchen." At first, Mom was confused
by my grandmother's words, but she began to go along
on her mother's visits, and she came to understand that
when people needed help, it was up to each of us to step
up to the plate and provide it.

"If you don't help," her mother would say, "you're not
going to leave a better world than when you came in."

That philosophy translated into what my mother
taught Suzy and me. "If you can complain about something in the community, then by God, you can fix it."
That has been my mother's legacy to us: the joy of volunteering. She helped us understand that we were supposed
to fix what was wrong, not wait for government or some-
body else to do it first. Perhaps Rabbi Hillel defines our
responsibility as human beings best. He said, "If not me,
who? If not now, when?" So I guess my interest in volunteering came naturally. In fact, I first became a volunteer
at the ripe old age of six when Suzy and I put on the backyard equivalent of a Broadway show in our neighborhood to raise money for polio research and raised a grand

total of sixty-four dollars. Believe me, that was a lot of money in those days.

Most people today probably don't remember that polio was a deadly public health threat back in the fifties. It was a very scary time for parents and children. In our neighborhood, parents were extremely careful and cautious about where their children played. One summer, polio seemed to be everywhere, and everything seemed to shut down. We didn't go to the movies. We didn't go to the public swimming pool, and as the headlines got worse, Mom even ended our playtime in the little plastic wading pool in our backyard.

Children of people we knew were struck down, and as my mother describes it today, "We just felt helpless." But a tough challenge was all Ellie Goodman needed to get involved.

I can still hear her telling Suzy and me, "It's up to you to fix things that are wrong." We took her words to heart and decided to do something about polio, too. We would put on a variety show, and we recruited every one of the twenty-three children who lived in the neighborhood to join our cause. Using the garage as a backdrop, everybody had a part in the show. The ones who couldn't or wouldn't sing and dance had to go out and collect folding chairs for the audience to sit on.

Suzy and I were a regular pair of impresarios. I thought it was a great performance of singing and dancing by everyone involved, especially me. I loved getting up in front of the crowd and trying a little two-step while "belting" out a song. That afternoon, as the applause rang out, I was convinced that I was destined to be the next Shirley Temple. After the "curtain" came down, however, Suzy informed me that in the future, I should leave the singing to her.

I can still remember how proud we felt on the day the two of us marched down to the Polio Association to hand over our sixty-four-dollar contribution. With that little show, we learned how important it was to take on a big cause, but we learned something else. We learned that giving to others made us feel good. That's the wonderful thing about volunteering. You get so much more back from those you help than you ever thought possible. Senator John McCain captures it beautifully when he says, "Nothing is more liberating than to fight for a cause larger than yourself."

Each of us becomes a volunteer in our own way. For me, it was Suzy's death that compelled me to begin the Susan G. Komen Breast Cancer Foundation and, in an odd way, gave my life new meaning. I can tell you that neither of us dreamed that my promise to her would one day become an international movement. My mother has been my rock and my compass over the past twenty years of the Komen Foundation. She's encouraged me every step of the way and has always been there to help me shoulder my responsibilities. I couldn't have done it without her. We've come a long way since the day a handful of women sat in my living room and started the Komen Foundation.

But the Komen Foundation has never been about one person or even two or three. It has been about many hearts and minds joined together in a great battle against a terrible killer. When we began, however, we had a dream and not much more.

I can't begin to tell you how tough our first couple of years really were. Looking back, it's a wonder we ever got off the ground. I worked day and night trying to educate myself about breast cancer, raise money, find ways to heighten public awareness of breast cancer, and take tearful calls from newly-diagnosed women looking for a friend. Underlying everything I did, one question continued to haunt me: could one person, or a handful of people, really make a difference? As hard as those first years were, we were absolutely convinced that we could.

At first, we relied on the generosity of a few large donors. Our emphasis was on fundraising as we worked to raise the seed capital we needed to get our fledgling organization off the ground. At our first Komen fundraiser, a small luncheon at the polo grounds, we nearly drowned as a freak storm literally rained on our parade. But we didn't let a little (or, in this case, a lot of) water stop us. Our first year, we were able to award two research grants totaling $30,000. The next year, we held our first major fundraiser, the First Annual National Awards Luncheon featuring a very special guest, former First Lady Betty Ford. By the end of 1983, our $200 had become $150,000.

> *"Advances are made by those with at least a touch of irrational confidence in what they can do."*
> Joan L. Curcio

Komen was up and running with me as volunteer chairman, a part-time secretary, and now a real office instead of my guest room. But more than that, we had the money to fund more research and new educational efforts to reach women with our message of hope.

One of my favorite Komen events in those first years was an auction that we held at the Fairmont Hotel in Dallas. My friend Carolyn Williams worked furiously to put the event together targeting men in Dallas with a little breast cancer "education" in order to get a lot of their support. Translation: Get them to pony up some big contributions for a cause they needed to be concerned about. In one of the planning sessions, someone cracked an old joke. "The only difference between men and boys," she said, "is the price of their toys." We all howled and immediately knew we had the name of our auction— "Toys for Boys"! We would auction items that appealed to men, like antique cars, sports packages, wine, and cigars. Sharon McCutchin, one of Komen's hardest- and longest-working volunteers, recruited her husband, Jerry, to the cause. Jerry's daughter, Barbara, had been diagnosed with breast cancer at thirty-two so the Komen Foundation became a family affair for them. Suzy's doctor and mine, George Blumenschein, was Barbara's doctor, too. I'm happy to tell you that she is a breast cancer survivor today.

For the auction, Jerry donated a plane. He brought it to the Fairmont in pieces and reassembled it right there in the room. It was the first and last time an airplane graced the interior of the Fairmont. All of our "plotting" worked beautifully. That night the Komen Foundation raised almost one million dollars for breast cancer research, and we all had a lot of fun, too. Looking back, I believe that evening was one of the turning points in the war against breast cancer. We had money, and we had men on board. We knew we needed both. Komen was on the map.

It didn't take long for me to realize, however, that if Komen was going to succeed in its mission to eradicate breast cancer as a life-threatening disease, we had to turn our cause into something more than just another fundraising event, just another charity ball. But what should our model look like? We weren't selling a product. The numbers that mattered to us weren't profit margins, but literally matters of life and death—mortality numbers, incidence rates, and the odds of recurrence. But we *were* selling something: the dream of a world without breast cancer.

I was adamant that Komen operate with sound business practices—in the black with enough set aside to cover two grant cycles. That meant no capital left to afford a *paid* staff in the beginning. So, we recruited a band of angels to our cause instead: friends, experienced businesspeople, and others committed to the fight and willing to give advice, moral support, and money. They were great. Many of them are still involved today, and together, we found our model—a combination of cause-related marketing and grassroots activism—the Komen Foundation's brand of social entrepreneurship.

But if we were to have any hope of succeeding, we knew that we had to bring breast cancer out into the open. As I said earlier, we had to change both the clinical and cultural environment. We also had to create a market for our dream, and get corporate America on board. We began to talk about breast cancer to anyone who would listen. We talked to the media, especially media outlets targeting women. We talked to men, especially about the need for money. We found them often uncomfortable with the discussion; but sometimes, that worked to our advantage. The more uncomfortable they were, the faster they would write a check just to get rid of me. What they didn't know was that I would be back for more.

But raising money from a few big donors wasn't enough. To achieve our mission fully, we needed to raise the public's awareness of breast cancer and the life-and-death issues that went with it. We weren't creating another charity; we were creating a movement. That meant Komen needed a mechanism to carry its message to every town and city in America. We needed to recruit our own messengers of hope. That is how the Komen Race for the Cure® was born. When I came up with the idea of the Race, everybody—I mean everybody—thought I was crazy. Even my mother. Women wouldn't go out on a Saturday morning to run in a sweaty race through town, they argued. But I was undeterred.

Eight hundred women ran in the first Komen Race for the Cure® in Dallas in 1983. Twenty years later, hundreds of thousands of local Komen volunteers, who share our dream of a world without breast cancer, and believe as we do that teamwork will get us there, are still running. Through the Race, we have established more than 100 Komen Affiliates in towns and cities across America, which support hundreds of local breast cancer education, screening and treatment programs, particularly for medically underserved communities. In 2000 alone, over 1.3 million people participated in the Race Series. You have no idea what it means to me personally to see thousands of people, young and old, men and women of every color running together like a band of angels for Suzy's cause, their cause, and *our* cause. I almost expect them to sprout wings, and I have to believe that somehow, somewhere she feels the same.

As the Komen Race for the Cure® began to gain visibility and momentum, we propelled a new idea to bring business on board—cause-related marketing. Today, with corporate sponsors from Ford to Yoplait, Komen's cause-related marketing has become a corporate and philanthropic phenomenon. But it wasn't always that way.

My first recruitment trip to New York looking for corporate "angels" was a complete disaster. I came up with the idea of putting hang-tags and labels on women's products like intimate apparel and cosmetics to remind women to get mammograms. I thought it was a great idea. Nobody else did. I had doors slammed in my face. I was thrown out of offices. Executives told me breast cancer was "negative marketing." They didn't want to put a disease on their packaging. One *woman* executive with a cosmetics company actually told me, "Our customers are buying beauty. They're not buying fear."

You have to remember that in 1982, Ben and Jerry may have scooped their first scoop of "Chunky Monkey," but the concept of social entrepreneurship was nearly as foreign in the business world as women in the boardroom.

Very few corporations tied themselves publicly to social issues—particularly those that had the potential to make their customers uncomfortable in any way. And I was asking them to embrace an issue that wasn't even mentioned aloud at the time. Needless to say, it was a tough sell. But, one by one, more and more forward-thinking companies embraced this new marketing concept because they understood that it was the right thing to do . . . and good business, too. They understood that the marketplace, like the workplace, was changing. Women were becoming an economic force to be reckoned with, and we were giving them an opportunity to reach women through their hearts

"To love what you do and feel that it matters—how could anything be more fun?"

Katherine Graham

and minds along with their pocketbooks. And to do the right thing at the same time.

Today, companies like Yoplait, New Balance, Johnson & Johnson, Ford, American Airlines, BMW, the Kellogg Company, Bristol-Myers Squibb, Hallmark, Wyndham and Lee have joined the Komen cause. These and so many other companies share our commitment and passion for increasing awareness of breast cancer and finding a cure.

In those early years, however, our most important conversation was with the women of America because sometimes we are our own worst enemy. Back then, women needed to understand the importance of early detection and of taking control of their own lives. They needed to understand that it was okay to talk openly about breast cancer, and they needed to believe that they had the power to do something about it.

It has been twenty years since the Komen Foundation began its conversation about breast cancer with the American people. Over those years, I have watched the

Foundation grow from its tiny beginning to what it is today—the nation's leading catalyst in the fight against breast cancer. The Foundation has more than 70,000 volunteers working through a network of more than one hundred U.S. and a growing number of international Affiliates, making it one of the most progressive grassroots organizations in breast cancer today. I used to wonder if one person could make a difference. I don't wonder any longer, but instead marvel at what can be done by first one person, then two, then ten, then thousands. Each and every contribution along the way, whether of time, talent, or money, has made a difference in the lives of women, like my sister and me, who have had to hear those terrible words, "I'm sorry, but it's breast cancer."

How far have we come toward making Suzy's dream a reality? I'm a natural born-sprinter, not a marathoner, so I like to see results yesterday. I won't be satisfied until breast cancer is no longer a threat to any woman, anywhere. We are still racing for the cure, but I believe the finish line is in sight. Let me tell you why by giving you a small glimpse of the wonderful progress that we have made over the past twenty years.

THE KOMEN FOUNDATION TODAY

The primary mission of the Susan G. Komen Breast Cancer Foundation is *to eradicate breast cancer as a life-threatening disease by advancing research, education, screening, and treatment.* To that end, literally hundreds of thousands of dedicated volunteers, complemented by a small Foundation staff, work tirelessly year after year to fulfill that mission.

Affiliates

When we began the Komen Foundation, we started in a fairly traditional way—holding dinners and luncheons to raise money to support a number of research grants. It didn't take long for us to realize, however, that we needed a different kind of structure because we had to do more than raise money. We had to change current attitudes toward breast cancer. Our answer was to create something that had never been attempted before—a grassroots network of committed volunteers—the Komen Foundation Affiliate Network.

Our first Affiliates began in Dallas and Peoria, followed by Wichita. Today, that number has grown to more than one hundred across the country. Inspired by my family's experience, each of these Affiliates has its own story to tell in terms of its founding. In some cities, it was the Junior League or other service organization that spearheaded the effort. In other places, it was the National Council of Jewish Women or groups of health care professionals or survivors joining together to "do something about breast cancer." For many communities, a Komen Race for the Cure® event was the impetus that led to a full-fledged Affiliate.

The genesis for each Affiliate is different, but they all share one thing. The women and men who create and sustain our Affiliates are our soldiers on the frontlines in the fight against breast cancer. They are what make the Komen Foundation unique among charitable health care organizations. At the Komen Foundation, our strength lies in our grassroots approach

Affiliate volunteers—our angel evangelists—are committed to funding crucial research and bringing needed breast health services to help the medically underserved in their communities. In 2000, Komen Affiliates awarded grants to hundreds of community-based breast health education, screening and treatment programs, along with support for innovative research like local clinical trials.

Experience taught us early that when it comes to health care and other social services, money often can be wasted through duplication of efforts. At the Komen Foundation, we knew that we didn't have a dime to waste. Our Komen Affiliates work closely with local medical experts and community leaders to conduct comprehensive community needs assessments in order to ensure that Affiliate funding supports only non-duplicative programs and services. Our job is to fill in the gaps. That, too, makes us unique as we work with other nonprofits, educational institutions, and government agencies to bring life-saving services to women who might otherwise fall through the cracks.

What also makes the Komen Affiliates Network stand out is our decision to keep most of the funds raised—up to 75 percent—in local communities. So, when you see a Komen Race for the Cure® event, you'll know that three-fourths of your donation stays where we believe it belongs—at the local level where the problems lie. The other 25 percent directly supports the Komen Foundation National Research Grant Program.

The Komen Affiliate Network has given the Foundation the ability to impact the lives of people in a very direct way. It has given us a conduit to get our message of hope out to people in local communities, changing their attitudes in ways that simply couldn't be done at the national level only. It has made breast cancer a "movement," which carries with it the power to influence those who make health care funding decisions at every level of government.

Grassroots activism is at the heart of the Komen Foundation's success whether it's our research, education, outreach, or advocacy efforts. And I am grateful every day for the thousands of Komen angels whose passion for this cause is changing the odds for millions of women around the world.

If you are interested in joining an Affiliate or creating one in your hometown, we'd love to help you get your "wings." (See the list of Affiliates and contact numbers at the end of this chapter.)

Research

Research holds the key to the cure of this devastating disease. We all know that. We also know that the Foundation's National Research Grant Program is often the only source of funding for cutting-edge research and for some of our youngest and most creative scientists.

Our investments in the future are clearly beginning to pay off, but it's important to remember that many of the breakthroughs that are making headlines today are the result of Komen's twenty-year history of support for crucial research. The Komen Foundation and its Affiliates will have raised an amazing $400 million by its twentieth birthday. Its National Research Grant Program has awarded more than 583 grants to institutions worldwide totaling more than $68 million for breast cancer research. Our Foundation currently supports research at many hospitals, universities, and clinics in the United States and around the world and remains one of the largest private sources of funding for breast cancer research and community outreach programs.

The Foundation's National Research Grant Program is regarded as one of the most innovative and responsive grant programs in breast cancer today, much of which has led to landmark discoveries such as the BRCA1 gene. In this research, for example, scientists were able to identify the gene that, when mutated, may increase a woman's risk of developing breast or ovarian cancer.

I'm particularly proud that our National Research Grants Program has been credited with bringing a new level of integrity to the grant application and review process. Komen's program adheres to a blind, peer-review process that is recognized by the National Cancer Institute (NCI) as a model for objectively funding basic, clinical and translational research.

Komen's current research grant portfolio includes:

- ✗ Training grants to doctoral dissertation students and postdoctoral fellows in order to recruit and retain young scientists in the field of breast cancer research;
- ✗ Basic, clinical and translational grants that encompass a broad number of focus areas including detection, diagnosis, prognosis, risk and prevention, treatment, tumor cell biology, and complementary and alternative medicines.
- ✗ Imaging technology research to improve breast cancer screening, diagnosis, and prognosis.
- ✗ Epidemiological research to address the disparities that exist in breast cancer incidence and mortality rates among specific populations.

I can't begin to tell you of all the specific fascinating research, both basic and clinical, that we are funding at major institutions across the country. But I can tell you this: We will not stop until a cure is found. We are determined to continue supporting scientists and researchers in the future because we believe that the day when breast cancer will be both preventable and curable isn't far away.

And what a day that will be when we can write the final chapter of this Foundation because research has found the cure we have dreamed of for more than twenty years.

Komen Race for the Cure®

By any measurement, our Komen Race for the Cure® Series, which originated in Dallas in 1983, has been a remarkable financial success, but it has also fundamentally changed our culture. People from all walks of life have joined in the fight from U. S. presidents to

Hollywood celebrities and some of the biggest names in the fashion industry. Pink ribbons symbolize our movement, and today corporations put them on everything from tennis shoes to golf balls to our favorite foods.

The Komen Race for the Cure® brought the fight against breast cancer out of the shadows and into the streets. It has grown from that first local Race to a national series of over a hundred Races with over one million participants annually, becoming the largest series of 5K runs/walks in the world. And it is still growing.

Francie Larrieu-Smith, five-time Olympian, has been the one and only National Honorary Chair of the Komen Race for the Cure® Series for a number of years. Our National Race, which takes place every year in Washington, D.C., has had its own stellar list of honorary chairs including the first chair, Marilyn Tucker Quayle. Over the years, the vice president and his wife have traditionally served in that capacity, and the tradition has been passed down from administration to administration. Former Vice President Al Gore and Tipper have always been two of our biggest supporters in Washington. President George W. Bush and Laura were Komen angels for many years in Texas before breaking with tradition in 2001 to become the first president and first lady to become honorary chairs of the National Race.

Along with being a road race for serious runners, the Komen Race for the Cure® Series is an emotionally-charged event that attracts many first-time and recreational runners and walkers. Participants include the young and old, those participating "in honor" or "in memory" of friends and family members, and especially those wonderful "survivors" donning pink caps, and T-shirts. They are an inspiration to us and to each other. They are why we do what we do at Komen.

We created the Race because we knew that Komen supporters wanted to do more than just contribute money. They wanted to feel they were really doing something about breast cancer in a more direct and personal way. We've found that the Race energizes local communities, raising awareness of breast cancer issues like the importance of early detection. Up to 75 percent of money raised stays in the local communities to support breast cancer education, screening, and treatment projects.

A minimum of 25 percent of the net Race proceeds goes to support Komen's National Research and Educational Grant Programs. For the past twenty years, these programs have provided much-needed funding for groundbreaking breast cancer research and for innovative projects in the areas of breast health education and breast cancer screening and treatment.

The Komen Race for the Cure® is an enormously effective way to communicate the message that most women don't have to die from breast cancer if they have the knowledge and the ability to access screening methods to detect breast cancer at its earliest stages. It is supported by generous, committed national partners, local sponsors, and by the countless volunteers who make it all work. For the latest information on the Komen Race for the Cure® Series, contact the automated Race Hotline at 1-888-603-RACE (1-888-603-7223) or visit www.raceforthecure.com.

Education

Until a cure is found, early detection is the most effective approach to breast cancer, and the key to early detection is making sure that women understand the importance of screening. Education empowers women to take charge of their own breast health, and that educational process is one of Komen's top priorities. One of our first major education efforts was the "Women's Leadership Summit on Mammography" that the Komen Foundation and the National Cancer Institute sponsored jointly in 1989. The Mammography Summit kicked off a national breast cancer screening drive, and we were privileged to have then-First Lady Barbara Bush rally the troops to "get the word out" as she spoke to more than 200 leaders of women's organizations attending. Today, through its Affiliate network, the Komen Foundation sponsors educational activities to help women understand the importance of breast health and to help cope when the disease has been diagnosed. We sponsor breast health seminars, training sessions, and media events year-round and all around the country. We also offer a wide range of printed materials through our Affiliates and from our national headquarters in Dallas. Breast health education is a woman's first line of defense.

When a woman learns she has breast cancer, the effects are devastating, but her family and friends pay a price, too. Our Komen Affiliates have done a remarkable job developing innovative programs that address not only the needs of the breast cancer patient, but the needs of the family as well. The Foundation is a trusted source of breast health and breast cancer information for people all over the world. Take advantage of Komen's resources that can help you in your fight against breast cancer. The Foundation's award-winning website, www.breastcancerinfo.com, provides up-to-the-minute information about research findings, clinical trials, local outreach programs, volunteer opportunities, Komen programs and events and much, much more. In addition, the Foundation operates a National Toll-Free Breast Care Helpline, 1 800 I'M AWARE®, that is staffed by trained, caring volunteers whose lives have been personally touched by breast cancer.

Along with our educational efforts year-round, every October during National Breast Cancer Awareness

Month we blanket radio, TV, and print media with information, special interest stories, facts, special promotions, public service announcements, and anything else that we can think of to help educate the public. Many corporations and organizations today recognize the importance of focusing attention on the issue of breast cancer, and we partner with them to create events that will help educate women and men on the importance of early detection. Many physicians and healthcare facilities across the country offer no-cost or low-cost mammography to qualified candidates on National Mammography Day and throughout the year.

Outreach

One of the primary goals of the Komen Foundation is to focus attention and resources on the critical problem of breast cancer in priority populations and the medically underserved. Special emphasis is placed on developing and funding outreach programs for these groups where the mortality rate is high. There are so many examples of important programs the Komen Foundation has funded to bring education, screening and treatment programs to the medically underserved, but two really stand out. The Witness Project® is a joint effort with the University of Arkansas Cancer Research Center. This national program enlists African-American breast cancer survivors to share their stories with other African-American women where they feel most at ease with themselves—their local churches. As you will see in chapter 12, sharing your feelings and experiences with breast cancer can help both you and others understand and deal with this difficult disease.

The "Patient Navigator" program is a pilot program designed to assist cancer patients and those at high risk by breaking down the institutional barriers to diagnostic and treatment services in a public hospital system. It was created at New York's Harlem Hospital by the director of the Cancer Control Center of Harlem, Dr. Harold P. Freeman.

As I have shared with you in this book, getting through the maze of paperwork, options, decisions, and other problems associated with breast cancer is overwhelming. And I was an educated breast cancer patient! Through this program, trained "patient navigators" volunteer to work one-on-one with patients to guide them through all phases of diagnosis and treatment. This pilot program has proven to be a highly effective and efficient system that is being used as a model in other hospitals across the country.

We continue to produce breast health materials in a variety of languages and materials targeted to priority populations such as Hispanics, African-Americans, Asians, Native Americans and Lesbians/Women Who Partner With Women. We are currently developing a breast health booklet for Arab women and their families. Our Affiliates and local grantees continue to produce materials in Russian, Arabic, Hebrew, Spanish, and many Asian dialects. We expect to launch our priority populations database in early 2002. This website will serve as a clearinghouse of grassroots breast health materials available for priority populations throughout the nation.

In 1998, the African-American National Advisory Council (AANAC) was formed to provide guidance and advice to help the Foundation address the specific breast health needs of African-American women. A number of outstanding and dedicated African-American women who have experience and expertise in the field of breast health and breast cancer comprise the council. We hope that the AANAC will serve as a model committee for other priority population advisory committees to be formed in the future. This is an area where much is left to be done.

In cooperation with the Centers for Disease Control (CDC), the Komen Foundation developed a model breast health outreach program for Hispanic women over the age of fifty entitled *La Salud de los Sensos y Usted* (Breast Health and You). This program coordinates Komen's educational outreach with existing state and local programs to increase the number of Hispanic women over fifty participating in breast and cervical screening programs. Special materials were produced in Spanish, and the program is staffed by trained volunteers.

Advocacy

I've worn a lot of hats over the past twenty years (even long after chemotherapy)—wife, mother, business-woman, author. But professionally, I might be best described as a "take-no-prisoners patient advocate." That's how I see myself. I refuse to let anyone or anything get in the way of my mission: a world without breast cancer.

Patient advocacy is one of the most important priorities of the Komen Foundation as well. In the early years of the Foundation, our focus was on raising the funds we needed to get the organization off the ground and begin to provide support for cutting-edge research. As our mission expanded, it included education, screening, and treatment, especially through Komen's Affiliates. Now, we find ourselves embracing the role of patient advocate more and more.

It didn't take long for us to realize that if we were to be successful in that mission, we needed to forge strong links with government at the federal, state, and local levels and provide our governmental representatives with a better understanding of breast cancer and the issues surrounding it.

Increased funding for breast cancer research was (and still is) one of our first priorities, and we knew that we had a big education job ahead of us. When the Komen Foundation was established, the federal government was only beginning to recognize the importance of funding breast cancer programs. In 1983, the federal budget for breast cancer research at the National Cancer Institute was $33 million. By 2002, the federal government will spend more than $766 million to fund breast cancer research, education, screening, and treatment programs.

The Komen Foundation has been a leader in the push to increase the budget of the National Institutes of Health where breakthrough cancer research in key areas such as biotechnology offers hope for all cancer survivors. But our advocacy programs extend far beyond federal funding issues. The Foundation plays a key role in educating legislators on the needs and concerns of breast cancer patients and survivors. One of our first successes was the passage of federal legislation that required all screening facilities, equipment and technicians be fully accredited in order to help ensure the quality and accuracy of mammograms. This activist role has earned the Foundation credibility with our political leadership that allows us to effectively speak out on behalf of everyone stricken by this disease. I have testified many times before Congress on breast cancer issues, and I'm pleased to be able to say that attitudes toward breast cancer have changed dramatically over the years.

The Komen Foundation was a driving force in support of the effort to create the Breast Cancer Research Stamp first issued in 1998. This stamp has not only raised public awareness of breast cancer significantly, it has also raised millions of dollars for breast cancer research.

We have also met with key Congressional leaders to urge continued strong federal support for the National Breast and Cervical Cancer Early Detection Program. This program provides screening, outreach and case-management services to assist high-risk, low-income women in all fifty states who otherwise do not have access to health care. At publication, more than one million women have been screened and thousands of breast and cervical cancers have been diagnosed. And yet, we still only reach about 15 percent of all eligible women. With increased funding, many more women will have access to this life-saving program.

Increasing participation in clinical trials has been one of the Komen Foundation's top public policy initiatives in recent years. Clinical trials are the only way to translate theoretical research progress into real cancer therapies; and for many patients, they offer the best treatment available. Unfortunately, only a tiny percentage of women with breast cancer today are participating in clinical trials that might save not only their own lives but also millions of others stricken with breast cancer in the future.

Too many barriers from fear to cost to geography keep too many people out of clinical trials, inhibiting promising research and slowing down our search for a cure. Many older cancer patients have worried that Medicare wouldn't cover routine patient care costs associated with clinical trials. On June 7, 2000, after a major patient advocacy effort among a number of health care organizations including the Komen Foundation, President Clinton issued an Executive Memorandum mandating that Medicare pay for patient care and treatment costs for patients enrolled in clinical trials.

As far as we've come in working to further the progress of the breast cancer movement, many issues still remain on the horizon. In the years ahead, the Komen Foundation will continue its work to break down the many barriers to clinical trials that still remain. We're tackling the touchy issue of patient privacy and the disclosure of personal health information. The Foundation will continue its effort to increase funding of breast cancer research, education, and screening programs as well as to support a patients' bill of rights.

Through a landmark research study, the Komen Foundation has also joined with the American Society of Clinical Oncology, Harvard and the Rand Corporation to address the serious lack of information about the quality of care cancer patients receive. This is one of the most important and innovative research projects that the Komen Foundation has funded in its nearly twenty-year history. By using a unique qualitative and quantitative approach, linking medical records to patient interviews, we will gather information crucial to developing a national, quality cancer care system. While this is a research study, the knowledge we gain will be invaluable to our patient advocacy efforts in the future.

One of the most extraordinary moments in the twenty-year history of the Komen Foundation took place on June 1, 2001, when President George W. Bush, one of the Foundation's long-time supporters, hosted a meeting at the White House with leaders in the breast cancer movement. The president invited a number of breast cancer experts including physicians, scientists, advocates, and survivors for a roundtable discussion on a range of breast cancer and health care delivery issues. We talked about the need to maintain research funding within government agencies. We raised the issue of expanding specialist education opportunities, both within medical training programs and continued medical education to ensure access to breast cancer specialists for all women. And we told him of the need to streamline the reimbursement paperwork burden for physicians and

TAKING CHARGE OF BREAST CANCER

create expanded access mechanisms to ensure that the newer targeted biological innovations are available quickly to patients for whom other treatment options have been exhausted. It was a great session followed by a very special reception in the beautiful and historic East Room of the White House.

The president invited several hundred breast cancer survivors who were participating in the Komen National Race for the Cure® the next morning to be his guests. Many of my fellow survivors wore pink survivors' T-shirts that might have seemed out of place on another day in this very formal room. But not on this day. I couldn't help but think we were making some history of our own.

The president, Mrs. Bush and Secretary of Health and Human Services Tommy Thompson all wore pink ribbons as the president told the Komen volunteers, "For the first time in human history we can say with some measure of confidence that the war on cancer is winnable."

Mrs. Bush, whose mother is a breast cancer survivor, spoke from the heart when she said, "As long as there is a reason to wear pink, my husband will be on our side." It was a day none of us will forget.

We have made so much progress since the days when Komen was just a handful of volunteers, and we've learned the effectiveness of volunteers in changing the hearts and minds of those in a position to help—whether it's the corporate world or the highest levels of our government. With survivor First Ladies Betty Ford and Nancy Reagan paving the way, Washington's doors are finally fully open to those advocating on behalf of breast cancer patients everywhere.

You can make a difference, too. Each of us has the ability and, I believe, the responsibility as citizens to talk to our representatives in Congress and at the state and local level about breast cancer. Keep yourself informed about key legislation in Congress that will impact the cause. Write letters, e-mail, or pick up the phone and make a call to your congressional representatives to register your individual support of these crucial efforts in the war against breast cancer.

As Ellie Goodman says, "We're all stewards of our country."

International

My duties as the founder of the Komen Foundation take me all over the world. On one of those trips to a country in Europe, someone showed me an obituary of a woman who had died recently of breast cancer. The newspaper never mentioned the actual cause of the woman's death. It said only that she had died of a "sad and lonely disease." I thought, if a newspaper could not tell the truth *after* her death, what kind of life must that woman have led as she fought her cancer?

In much of the world over the past century, women's health has never been a government or even a private sector priority. The United States was no different twenty years ago. To help change these outdated attitudes as we have done here, I've spent much of my time and efforts trying to extend the reach of the Komen Foundation to other countries around the world. Clearly, breast cancer knows no boundaries. It doesn't stop at our borders, so why should Komen's efforts to fight breast cancer end at the water's edge?

Through Komen's international initiatives, we hope to accelerate the pace of breast cancer awareness and the need for research funding around the globe so that what took twenty years to achieve here can be accomplished far sooner in other nations.

Recognizing the global impact of breast cancer and the value of coordinated advocacy in battling this disease, we have already launched Affiliates in Greece, Germany, and Italy, and others are soon to follow.

We have also already provided more than $1.9 million in funding for international breast cancer research in places as far away as Brisbane, Australia and Tel Aviv, Israel. Another $1.5 million has gone to support community education and outreach programs like Breast Cancer Awareness Day in Madrid, Spain. Komen funding has also supported a number of international conferences from Mexico to Japan.

But I always have a soft spot in my heart for the Race for the Cure.® In May 2000, the very first international Komen Race for the Cure® was held in Rome, Italy, where women are still hesitant to talk about their disease. The silent epidemic still goes on in most of the world. But more than 5,600 courageous women and men broke with tradition in one of the world's most traditional places—the Eternal City. They ran and walked in the footsteps of Caesar, in the shadow of the Coliseum, past the Forum and Circus Maximus through center-city Rome.

One of the Komen Race volunteers tells a wonderful story. Because people don't often talk about their illness in Italy, when the pink Komen survivor hats arrived from Komen headquarters, they didn't think there would be many takers. After the hats were unpacked and put on a table, one woman, a survivor who'd been helping out all week, quietly put a hat in her purse. Later, the volunteer saw her at the Race; and, by then, she was carrying it in her hand. But when she crossed the finish line, the woman was proudly wearing the hat that told everyone she had breast cancer and so did many of her fellow survivors. One person can make a difference.

No one exemplifies that more than Dr. Martina Lies, the co-chair of the first Komen Race for the Cure® in Germany. This woman is truly remarkable, not only for helping to put together the Race in less than a year, but also for devoting endless hours to community and survivor outreach establishing the Komen name in Germany in the process. She is a human dynamo, speaking to women in groups large and small—anywhere someone will listen to her message of the importance of early detection; convincing politicians, journalists, and pharmaceutical companies to get involved in the fight against breast cancer. And she does it all in an environment where women are not expected to talk about breast cancer.

It's déjà vu all over again for me hearing Dr. Lies' story. The first Komen Frankfurt Race for the Cure® was held in August 2000. Everyone told her it would never work. Well, thousands of runners and walkers proved the "experts" wrong. It was the third largest running event ever held in the region.

Seeing a Komen volunteer give her time, energy, heart, and soul to the fight against breast cancer is not so unusual. What sets Dr. Lies apart is the fact that she is not only a doctor, wife, and devoted mother of a three-year-old daughter, but she is battling the emotional and physical challenges of a patient with metatastic breast cancer. Dr. Lies was given the 2000 Komen Community Service award for individual contribution. It doesn't seem enough.

In 2001, our Athens Affiliate held its first Komen Greece Race for the Cure® in Athens, which was a remarkable event as well. There were more than four thousand registrants, yet only forty brave women dared to don the pink cap. Yes, there is a lot left to do. I can't tell you how exciting it is to see the enthusiasm and hope these new international Affiliates are generating for our cause in their home countries. They have become a part of the growing Komen family, and I am so proud that our efforts are not only changing our own world but the lives of women a world away.

As you can see, Komen is working on many, many fronts to battle this disease. But until a cure is found, the Komen Foundation will continue its fight for the right of every woman to live without the fear of breast cancer.

I was touched when I read a letter from a young woman by the name of Angela who had recently run in a Komen Race for the Cure.® She was thirteen when her mother was diagnosed with breast cancer. She was seventeen when she left school to take care of her mother full-time.

A month after Angela got married, breast cancer finally took her mother. Today, Angela is married with children, and she runs in memory of her mother. She wrote, "What an experience it is to know that I'm helping future generations find a cure and win this battle. One day, my children will not have this deep pit inside them every time they look in their children's eyes."

If the extraordinary work of the dedicated and caring people of Komen are an indication, I am convinced that Angela will get her wish. I know in my heart and my mind that major breakthroughs are near.

I hope this book will be helpful to you. But remember, information is a woman's best friend. So, share this book with someone else and become a part of the Komen family.

Contact us:

✗ for breast cancer information
✗ to receive our newsletter
✗ to volunteer
✗ for a list of Komen Affiliates and Komen Race for the Cure® Events
✗ to contribute to the cause

The Susan G. Komen Breast Cancer Foundation
Headquarters
5005 LBJ Freeway, Suite 250
Dallas, TX 75244

972-855-1600 Fax: 972-855-1605
Helpline: 1-800-I'M AWARE®
Website: www.breastcancerinfo.com

Komen Affiliate Network

The Komen Foundation has more than 70,000 volunteers working through a network of over 110 U.S. and a growing number of international Affiliates.

Please call our 1 800 I'M AWARE® Helpline to learn how you can join in the activities in a city near you.

2001 Komen Affiliate Locations

Alabama:	Birmingham		
Arkansas:	Fayetteville	Little Rock	
Arizona:	Phoenix	Tucson	
California:	Fresno	Los Angeles	Orange County
	Sacramento	San Diego	San Francisco
	Temecula		
Colorado:	Aspen	Colorado Springs	
	Denver	Greeley	
Connecticut:	New Britain		
Florida:	Daytona	Jacksonville	Miami
	Tampa Bay	West Palm Beach	
Georgia:	Atlanta	Macon	
Hawaii:	Honolulu		
Iowa:	Davenport	Des Moines	Ottumwa
Idaho:	Boise	Coeur d'Alene	
Illinois:	Bloomington	Chicago	Decatur
	Peoria		
Indiana:	Evansville	Indianapolis	Terre Haute
Kansas:	Wichita		
Kentucky:	Lexington	Louisville	
Louisiana:	Baton Rouge	Lafayette	Monroe
	New Orleans	Shreveport	Thibodaux
Massachusetts:	Boston		
Maryland:	Baltimore		
Maine:	Bangor		

Michigan:	Battle Creek	Detroit	Grand Rapids
	Lansing		
Minnesota:	Brainerd	Minneapolis	
Missouri:	Joplin	Kansas City	St. Louis
Mississippi:	Jackson	Tupelo	
Montana:	Helena		
North Carolina:	Charlotte	Lenoir	Raleigh
	Winston-Salem		
Nebraska:	Omaha		
New Jersey:	Princeton	North Jersey	
New Mexico:	Albuquerque		
Nevada:	Las Vegas	Reno	
New York:	Albany	Buffalo	Elmira
	Syracuse	New York	
Ohio:	Cincinnati	Cleveland	Columbus
	Toledo		
Oklahoma:	Oklahoma City	Tulsa	
Oregon:	Portland		
Pennsylvania:	Philadelphia	Pittsburgh	Scranton
Rhode Island:	Providence		
South Carolina:	Charleston	Greenville	
Tennessee:	Chattanooga	Knoxville	Memphis
	Nashville		
Texas:	Amarillo	Austin	Central Texas
	Dallas	El Paso	Houston
	Lubbock	Plano	Fort Worth
	San Antonio	Texarkana	Tyler
	Wichita Falls		
Utah:	Salt Lake City		
Virginia:	Richmond	Tidewater	
Vermont:	Manchester		
Washington:	Seattle		
Wisconsin:	Madison	Milwaukee	
West Virginia:	Charleston		
Wyoming:	Cheyenne		

Chapter Four
Breast Health
What Every Woman Should Know

"Some people think women are supposed to have a sixth sense. Listen, I don't even know what my birth sign is."
Lorraine Mintzyer

For Suzy, who grew up in the era when Marilyn Monroe was touted as the perfect woman, having a curvaceous figure was very important. Tight sweaters were all the rage back then, and she was very much aware that her good looks were credited to more than just a pretty face. Although there was only a three-year difference in our ages, Suzy and I were on the tail end of one era and the beginning of another totally different era as far as what was in vogue when we entered our adult lives. While my sister and her friends were striving for a look of voluptuous femininity, my friends and I believed that "thin was in." Twiggy was our idol, and we strove for a look of slender elegance. For Suzy and me, the timing of the fashion trends was ideal. She was shorter than I am, about five feet five inches, and although she was never overweight, her figure was just like an hourglass. By the time I reached college, my height had caught up to my body weight; and at almost six feet, I was tall and thin. Suzy and I literally didn't see eye-to-eye on what constituted the perfect female figure; but regardless of our differences, our individual self-images were extremely important and personal to us.

Diagram of a Healthy Breast

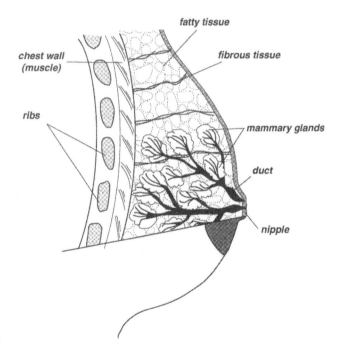

The importance of a woman's breasts to her total sexuality is imbedded deeply in her mind at a very tender
age. This happens long before a young girl can even begin
to fathom the real physiological purpose of her breasts,
which is, of course, to feed her babies. Although her
maternal instincts are often nurtured in childhood
through the use of dolls, those dolls come with a pretend
bottle to complete the fantasy. Today, it may be likely
that a young girl will have the opportunity to watch her
mother breast-feed a younger sibling. But when Suzy
and I were growing up, most children were bottle-fed;
consequently, many women of our generation never
fully understood that breasts were more than sexual
objects. I know I didn't.

Back then, teenagers took "health class," the precur-
sor to today's sex education. Ironically, what little was
taught about health focused on menstruation, inter-
course, and pregnancy; not on our breasts, much less on
our breast health. Teenagers today are far more sophisticated on these subjects thanks to sex education, but
many are still embarrassed by the subject and reluctant
to ask questions in front of their peers.

The point is that it is not uncommon for a woman to
enter adulthood having little more knowledge about her
breasts than her cup size. In order for any of us to truly
understand breast cancer, we must first understand the
basic anatomy of the breasts and how they function.

BREAST HEALTH BASICS

Breasts are glandular organs, physiologically designed
for one particular purpose: to produce milk. Your
breasts will go through many natural changes from
puberty through menopause. And, like most women,
you may experience some common breast changes at
some point in your life. The normal cycle of female

hormones affects both the outward appearance and the inside structure of the breasts. By understanding these normal changes as they occur, you will be better able to recognize any *unusual* changes that could be warning signals for potential problems. But even if you *never* have a problem, it is important to know what is happening to your body. It is no longer acceptable for women merely to go along for the ride where our health is concerned. We need to be in the driver's seat *with* the road map. We have been content, in the past, to turn our bodies over to our physicians unconditionally as soon as *they* point out the first sign of trouble. Too often, women wait until they feel pain before they go to their physicians. With breast cancer, this can be too late, for in its early stages it usually causes no pain.

> *"I was raised in a small town called Critz [Virginia]. It was so small that our school taught Driver's Ed and Sex Ed in the same car."*
> Mary Sue Terry

But this is a new era in health care. With routine checkups, problems can be identified early when they are most easily treated. By knowing how our bodies are supposed to be functioning, we can use the medical profession to support our wellness rather than merely to treat our illness.

It is also crucial for a woman to understand the physiology of her breasts, as well as their anatomical structure, because of the close proximity of the breasts to other vital organs such as the heart, lungs, and liver. (Although a man's breasts are located in the same place, their mass, weight, and function do not have the same impact on the body.) Each woman's breasts are unique in size and shape. The differences are based on one's heredity and total body weight. Cosmetic reconstructive surgery must also be considered a variable today because of its growing popularity. Many women have breast enlargements to make them feel more feminine and attractive, while others try to improve their self-image by having breast reductions.

Most of us realize that breast size varies, but there are other differences as well. Nipples and the areolas may also vary in color and appearance. Some women might have small hairs and/or bumps around the areola; others might be smooth and clear. These differences are normal and are nothing to worry about.

If you could look underneath the skin and see how the breast is structured, it would look very much like the diagram on page 100. Your breast tissue begins just below the collarbone and extends from the armpit to the breast-bone and down to the bra line. Breasts are made up of lobules, ducts, connective tissue, lymph nodes, muscles, and fat.

The first changes in our breasts occur during puberty as breast tissue develops and our breasts grow larger. During pregnancy and after childbirth, milk is produced in the lobules and carried through the ducts to the nipple openings. Our breasts increase in size during this time.

As we age and enter menopause, our ovaries stop producing hormones and the number of lobules decreases. As a result, we lose breast tissue and the size and shape of your breasts change. Much of the more dense breast tissue is replaced with fat. We all know this process; unfortunately, isn't limited to the breasts and is a fact of life for all of us as we age.

Breast terminology can be confusing. It was for me at first. So, before we go any farther, here are some short explanations of terms you need to know.

☒ *Lymph nodes:* Glands that produce white blood cells that fight bacteria and toxins. Fluids from the breast drain primarily to lymph node chains located under the arm. At the underarm, axillary lymph nodes become quite important in breast cancer because they are one of the first regions where cancer can spread.

- ℛ *Fibrous tissue:* Extends from just beneath the surface of the skin to the chest wall muscles to provide support for the breast. It also separates the breast into segments. Younger women have much more dense, fibrous tissue, allowing for firmer breasts.
- ℛ *Mammary glands and ductal system:* The mammary glands are the milk-producing glands. During pregnancy, milk is produced in the fifteen to twenty separate lobes of each gland and is carried through ducts to the nipples during breast feeding. The ductal system drains milk from the mammary glands to the nipple. Each ductal pattern is unique, like a fingerprint.
- ℛ *Fat tissue:* This tissue forms a covering for the fibrous tissue. The amount of fat varies according to a woman's weight and age. After menopause, the mammary glands begin to shrink and are replaced by fat, causing the breasts to lose their firmness.
- ℛ *Nipple and areola:* The nipple sticks out from the breast. The ducts that carry milk from the mammary glands lead to the nipple, from which the milk is drawn by a nursing baby. The areola is the dark area of skin surrounding the nipple.
- ℛ *The chest wall:* consists of the ribs and a large group of muscles that fan over them. These muscles and ribs form the firm background onto which the breast is attached.

Common Breast Changes

Your breasts will go through many natural changes from puberty through menopause. And, like most women, you may experience some common breast changes at some point in your life. These conditions might include lumps, pain, and nipple discharge.

The good news is that most of these changes are both common and benign (non-cancerous). For instance, do your breasts feel swollen and tender before your period? If so, you might be experiencing cyclic breast change—a breast condition that affects about half of all women. Cyclic breast changes are related to the menstrual cycle. That's because your breast tissue is directly influenced by the same hormones that affect your period: estrogen and progesterone.

Your breasts may even feel tender and heavy. Lumps form when extra fluid collects in the breast. These are normal changes. Both lumps and swelling generally go away by the end of your period. It's a good idea to inform your health care provider about any—even common—changes.

Let's take a look at some other common breast conditions.

- ✗ *Cysts*: Fluid-filled sacs in the breast tissue. They most often occur in women in their thirties and older. Cysts are almost always harmless.
- ✗ *Fat Necrosis*: This refers to the firm lumps formed by damaged fatty tissue. They can develop as a result of a bruise or a blow to the chest. These lumps are more likely to form in women who are overweight.
- ✗ *Fibroadenomas:* Round, rubbery, benign tumors. Fibroadenomas are the most common tumors found in women in their late teens and early twenties. Although these tumors are not cancerous, they may grow larger with pregnancy or when a woman is breast-feeding.
- ✗ *Fibrocystic Breasts:* Fibrocystic breast change is lumpiness plus tenderness or pain at certain times of the month. The lumpiness may become more obvious as you approach middle age.
- ✗ *Sclerosing Adenosis:* A condition that involves excessive growth of the fibrous tissue and the lobules. The growth uncommonly causes breast pain. It may even produce lumps.
- ✗ *Nipple Discharge*: A secretion of liquid from the nipple. Take note of the color and texture of the discharge in order to let your doctor know. Nipple discharge may be of concern if it appears spontaneously

without squeezing the nipple, if it is in one nipple only, or if it is bloody. Your health care provider may take a sample of the discharge and send it to a laboratory to be tested.

✗ *Non-Cyclical Breast Pain*: Often experienced in one specific area of the breast. This kind of non-cyclical pain is not related to your hormones or monthly periods and does not vary over your monthly cycle. If you experience this type of pain, you should see a trained medical professional.

✗ *Non-Breast Origin Pain*: Usually starts in the chest or ribs. If you have this kind of pain, it may not be a breast condition at all. It may be another medical problem that should be checked by a trained medical professional.

Though not life-threatening, benign breast changes can be distressing for a woman. Talk to your physician or health care provider about how these breast changes can be treated. Your physician may recommend surgically removing fibroadenomas, fat necrosis, and sclerosing adenosis, or draining a cyst.

There are also things you can do to relieve some types of changes. To treat fibrocystic breast changes, physicians may recommend wearing a well-fitted support bra to hold the breasts close to the chest. Eating a balanced diet providing all of the vitamins like E and B6 may also help relieve or prevent breast pain and changes.

What Can I Do?

The same three processes that tell you what is normal for your breasts—breast self-examination, clinical breast exam, and screening mammography—are also the best possible methods widely available for finding problems in your breasts. Before discussing these methods, however, I want to stress that not all breast abnormalities are cancerous. Hundreds of thousands of women experience a breast lump or other abnormalities at some time in their lives and never have cancer. So, if an abnormality appears, don't panic, but do make an appointment to see your physician. Early detection and optimum treatment offer the best chance of surviving breast cancer. When breast cancer is confined to the breast, the 5-year survival rate is over 95 percent.

So, how do you begin to take charge of your own breast health? Faithfully follow this early detection plan.

Monthly Breast Self-Examination

Breast self-examination (BSE) is one of the most effective health habits a woman can acquire. Developing this habit is one way of taking charge of your body and becoming a responsible custodian of your own good health. A breast self-exam is an uncomplicated process to help you become familiar with the normal look and feel of your breasts. It requires only a few minutes of your time and should be done once a month just as your period is ending. If you are postmenopausal and no longer have monthly periods, do BSE on the same day each month. Pregnant women should examine their breasts the same day of each month, as should breast-feeding mothers. Nursing mothers should feed babies just before breast self-examination.

All women should perform monthly BSE by age twenty. Make BSE a time for relaxation and self-care. While at first it may feel awkward, the more times you do your BSE, the more comfortable and familiar with your breasts you will become. That familiarity could one day save your life. Here are the basic steps to do your Breast Self Exam:

☧ First, in front of a mirror, check for any changes in the shape or look of your breasts. Note any skin or nipple changes such as dimpling or nipple discharge. Inspect your breast in the following positions: arms at side, arms over head, hands on hips pressing firmly to flex chest muscles, and bending forward at the waist.

X Then, lie down on your back with a pillow under your right shoulder and place your right hand behind your head.

X Use the finger pads of your left hand to check your entire right breast, upper chest, nipple, and underarm area.

X Start under your arm, making small, dime-sized circles in an up and down pattern.

X Continue this pattern using light, medium, and firm pressure.

Repeat these steps on your left breast. When lying down, remember to put your left hand under your head and a pillow under your left shoulder.

If you notice any change in the normal look and feel of your breasts, make an appointment to see a trained medical professional. Explain that you are concerned about a breast change that you found while examining your breasts. Remember, most lumps are benign.

Write BSE on your calendar or day planner to remind yourself when to examine your breasts each month. Look for opportunities to remind your friends to do their BSE. You owe it to yourself, your family, and friends. Early detection saves lives!

Clinical Breast Exam (CBE)

In conjunction with your mammogram and breast self-exam, it is important to have a yearly clinical breast exam given by your health care provider. A small percentage of breast lumps that are not detected by mammography can be felt during a clinical breast examination. Therefore, it is very important that women have *both* a clinical breast examination and a screening mammogram performed. A physician who has been trained in breast examination is sensitive to abnormalities you and I might miss on our own, especially if we have been negligent in performing our monthly breast self-examinations. Your health care provider should perform the CBE during regular checkups.

We have made tremendous strides over the past twenty years in sensitizing physicians to the importance of breast health, but if your health care provider does not examine your breasts, ask for it. Or find one who does. Remember, you're in charge!

During the CBE, your health care provider will look for changes in the normal appearance of the breast such as size, shape, or color. Then, your health care provider will feel the entire breast area for new lumps. This is a good time to ask your doctor any questions or discuss any concerns that you might have about doing your BSE, common breast changes, or your risk profile (your chance of developing breast cancer).

The exam will consist of essentially the same procedure described in BSE. It should include a visual exam and palpation while sitting and lying down.

Make sure that your health care provider checks your breasts at least every three years if you are between the ages of twenty and thirty-nine, and every year after age forty.

Mammogram

In conjunction with BSE and CBE, a mammogram is the best screening tool widely available to detect breast cancer at its earliest, most treatable stages. A mammogram is an X-ray picture of the breast. It has the ability to detect breast cancers before they can be felt. The mammogram machine is designed to take pictures of the breasts. It uses a very small amount of X-ray radiation that is not harmful to you.

During the mammogram, your breasts are pressed between two plastic plates. This flattens the breast tissue so that the X ray will be clear. A specially trained radiologist

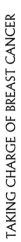

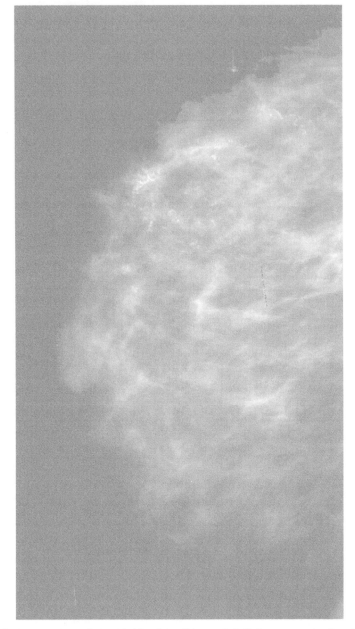

A mammogram is crucial in detecting and defining cancers of various sizes.

who looks for cancer or other breast changes reads the black and white X-ray pictures. The mammogram takes just a few minutes, and you will usually have your results within two weeks.

Starting at age forty, women should get a mammogram every year. If you are under forty and have a family history of breast cancer or other concerns about your personal risk, talk to your healthcare professional about a risk assessment and when to begin screening mammograms. Remember that some breast cancers are not detected by mammography but can be felt during clinical breast exam. So, it's important to have both—a clinical breast exam and a mammogram—done every year.

Warning Signs

If you notice a breast change—such as a new lump or thickening, nipple discharge, redness and swelling, or pain—don't ignore it! Make an appointment to see your doctor as soon as possible. It may be a harmless breast condition or it could be a warning sign for breast cancer. Believe me, worrying about what might or might not be cancer is worse than knowing. Let a trained medical professional make the diagnosis. Pay particularly close attention to the following warning signs:

- 𝖷 A new, hard lump or thickening of your breast tissue
- 𝖷 Change in the size or shape of your breast
- 𝖷 Dimpling or puckering of the skin on your breast
- 𝖷 Swelling, redness, or increased warmth of your breast
- 𝖷 Breast pain that does not vary with your monthly cycle
- 𝖷 Pulling in of your nipple
- 𝖷 An itchy, sore, or scaling area of your nipple
- 𝖷 Nipple discharge that starts suddenly

You should be aware of these warning signs because prompt attention could help you find breast cancer early when it is most treatable.

TAKING CHARGE OF BREAST CANCER

Knowing that mammography is currently the best method widely available to detect breast cancer, it is nothing less than horrifying to learn that still only 60 percent of all women over the age of fifty have a yearly screening mammogram. Yet, most women over the age of eighteen *have* had a gynecological exam. Why do you suppose a woman would be so conscientious about the health of one part of her body and negligent about the health of another? The answer is probably fear. Fear of hearing something she doesn't want to hear. Fear of losing a breast. Fear of abandonment by a loved one. And fear of losing her life.

But there is no need to be afraid. You should know that 80 percent of all breast abnormalities are not cancerous; and let me say it once again, when breast cancer is detected while confined to the breast, the 5-year survival rate is over 95 percent. More important, the likelihood of death from breast cancer is also dramatically decreased.

Another reason women are reluctant to get a mammogram is the expense. It can cost up to two hundred dollars for a mammogram. Most insurance programs, however, including Medicare, cover annual mammograms. There are also many free or low-cost screening programs available today, so take advantage of them if you lack insurance or financial resources. Call the Komen Foundation's National Toll-Free Breast Care Helpline at 1.800 I'M AWARE® for more information on breast health and breast cancer. The Helpline is answered by trained, caring volunteers whose lives have been personally touched by breast cancer.

Although an abnormality in your breast does not necessarily mean cancer, this does not mean you can ignore it or put off consulting your healthcare provider about it. Get a diagnosis as soon as possible. If it is cancer, catch it before it has a chance to spread.

Chapter Five
Understanding Your Risk for Breast Cancer

"Nothing in life is to be feared. It is only to be understood."
Madame Curie

H elen Hayes once joked that "the hardest years in a woman's life are those between 10 and 70." While most of us are perfectly happy to be female, our gender does have its occasional drawbacks. Simply being a woman and growing older puts you at risk for breast cancer. As a matter of fact, those are the two greatest risk factors for developing breast cancer.

AGE: A MAJOR FACTOR

A woman's chance of getting breast cancer increases with age. For a woman born today in the U.S., her risk by age 30 is 1 out of 2,525.

By age 40: 1 out of 217
By age 50: 1 out of 50
By age 60: 1 out of 24
By age 70: 1 out of 14
By age 80: 1 out of 10

But there are also a number of other factors that may impact your chances of getting the disease. Having several risk factors for breast cancer does not mean that you will get breast cancer. It just means that your chances of getting the disease are higher than women who have fewer risk factors. In fact, most women diagnosed with breast cancer have no known risk factor. So why do some women get breast cancer and others with similar factors don't? The causes are not yet fully understood. However, we do know that there are certain known risk factors—some that you can control and others that you cannot. In all likelihood, you will have more than one risk factor at some point in your life. But, remember, even if you do not have any of these risk factors, you can still develop breast cancer.

Factors you can change:

❊ Drinking more than one alcoholic drink per day. Numerous studies have shown that high levels of alcohol intake most likely increases the risk of breast cancer.

❊ Being overweight or gaining weight as an adult. The effect of adult weight on the risk of breast cancer is different among pre- and post-menopausal women. Before menopause, it appears that being somewhat overweight decreases a woman's risk of getting breast cancer. After menopause, however, being overweight increases the risk for the disease by about 20 to 60 percent. A very large study of U.S. nurses found that weight gained after age eighteen increases the risk of both developing and dying from breast cancer in postmenopausal women.

❊ Not getting regular exercise (at least three times a week for at least thirty minutes) Physical activity may protect you from breast cancer if you are premenopausal or are a younger postmenopausal woman. Exercise reduces estrogen levels, fights obesity, lowers insulin levels and boosts the immune system.

❊ Eating a non-healthy diet. For overall wellness and possibly to decrease your breast cancer risk, it is recommended that women consume a well-balanced diet rich in fruits and vegetables, whole grains and legumes.

❊ Taking birth control pills for five years or longer can slightly increase your risk. However, there is no apparent increase in a woman's risk of breast cancer ten or more years after she has stopped using oral contraceptives.

✂ Currently or recently using hormone replacement therapy (HRT) for ten years or longer may slightly increase your risk.

✂ Being exposed to large amounts of radiation frequently, such as having very frequent spinal X rays during scoliosis treatment.

Factors you cannot change:

✂ Getting older—the older you get, the greater your risk of breast cancer

✂ Having already had breast cancer

✂ Having certain mutated breast cancer genes (BRCA1 or BRCA2)

✂ Having had your first period before age twelve

✂ Having had no children

✂ Having had your first child after age thirty

✂ Having started menopause after fifty-five

✂ Having a mother, daughter, or sister who has had breast cancer.

✂ A history of a benign breast biopsy, especially a biopsy showing atypical hyperplasia, or carcinoma in situ

If you are a woman at higher than average risk, talk with your physician. There are options available, such as the following:

✂ Starting your yearly mammograms before the age of forty.

✂ Close monitoring of the breasts by having more frequent mammograms and breast exams.

✂ Taking an antiestrogen drug to help reduce the chance of getting breast cancer.

✂ Having a prophylactic or preventive mastectomy (removal of one or both breasts) to reduce the chance of getting breast cancer.

✗ Participating in a chemoprevention trial (research study of the effectiveness of drugs to prevent breast cancer). See the resource section of this book for the Physician Data Query (PDQ) contact information.

DIAGNOSING A BREAST CONDITION

First, you need to know the difference between screening and diagnosing a breast condition. A screening test is regularly performed when no unusual symptoms have occurred. A diagnostic test, on the other hand, is done after a suspicious condition has been found. If you notice a change in your breast that is abnormal, make an appointment to see your physician right away. He or she will perform a clinical breast exam (CBE) and may arrange for you to undergo diagnostic testing. This may include a diagnostic mammogram, ultrasound, and/or biopsy.

Diagnostic Mammogram

During a diagnostic mammogram, more pictures of the breast are taken in order to evaluate the breast area of concern. Each X-ray picture is compared to previous pictures (if they exist) to see if any changes have occurred. If the mammogram shows that further testing is needed, an ultrasound or biopsy may be recommended.

Ultrasound

An ultrasound exam generally can distinguish between a liquid-filled cyst and a solid lump in the breast. The technologist spreads a thin layer of gel over the breast; then guides a hand-held scanning device back and forth across the suspicious breast area. The device sends sound waves that will either pass through a cyst or bounce off a solid area. A computer converts the sound waves into a picture on a video monitor. The test is safe, painless, and uses no radiation. If it turns out that the lump is solid, your physician may then discuss biopsy options with you.

Biopsy

A biopsy involves removing a sample of breast tissue. During this procedure, the physician removes breast tissue using a needle (needle biopsy) or a scalpel (open biopsy). Then, the tissue is examined under a microscope to check for the presence of cancer or precancerous cells. The diagnostic method that your physician recommends will depend on your condition and general health. A biopsy is generally not painful because the breast is numbed, but you may feel some discomfort.

Needle Biopsy

Because it is fast and simple, this method is often done first. If your physician cannot feel the lump, special equipment is used to guide the needle to the lump.

Fine needle: A thin, hollow needle is used to remove a few cells from the breast lump. It can be done in the physician's office and only takes a few minutes.

Core needle: A thicker, hollow needle removes a larger amount of tissue. As with fine needle biopsy, a core needle biopsy is done for an abnormal area found by mammogram. Ultrasound or a stereotactic mammogram is needed to accurately guide the needle to the suspicious area. The skin is nicked with a scalpel so the needle can enter. This type of needle biopsy is done in a medical office, outpatient surgery center, or hospital.

Open Biopsy

An open biopsy uses surgical cutting to take out breast tissue. It is done in a hospital or outpatient surgery center. The procedure causes some bleeding, pain, and scarring. Most women are able to go home the same day.

Excisional: The entire lump plus some surrounding normal tissue is removed. This is the most common type of open biopsy and the most accurate way to diagnose breast cancer. It is sometimes called a *lumpectomy* or *partial mastectomy*. Although the primary purpose is to diagnose cancer, a biopsy can also be a surgical treatment to remove cancer.

Incisional: Only a portion of the lump is removed. It is most often done on women whose tumors are too large to be removed through excisional biopsy.

A biopsy is the only way to tell if a suspicious lump is cancerous. If the thought of a needle in your breast makes you a little queasy, relax! You're normal, and you're not alone. Most women do feel anxious and even depressed about needing a biopsy. I know I did. Try to ease your mind by reminding yourself that about 80 percent of all lumps that are biopsied turn out to be benign (non-cancerous), even among women whose problem was found through a mammogram. Everyone gets nervous, however, so bring a friend or family member along for support and to help drive you home.

Here are some questions to ask your physician:

- ✗ What type of biopsy do you recommend for me and why?
- ✗ Who will do the biopsy and how?
- ✗ How long will it take?
- ✗ How much of the tissue will be removed?
- ✗ What are the possible side effects?
- ✗ When and how will I get the results?
- ✗ If a problem is found, what will we do next? When?
- ✗ How soon will I be able to return to my normal routine?
- ✗ How visible will my scar be? Where will it be?
- ✗ How much will the test cost and will my insurance cover it?

NEW IMAGING METHODS

The fast pace of developing technology has given birth to a number of new and promising imaging methods to detect breast cancer. However, because they are new, they may not be in routine use. At present, they are used mainly in research studies and, sometimes, to get more information about a tumor found by another method. Each of these new methods generates a computerized image that a physician can analyze for the presence of an abnormal breast lump.

Scintigraphy

Also called *scintimammography*, this test uses a special camera to show where a tracer (a radioactive chemical) has adhered to a tumor. A scanner is then used to see if the breast lump has picked up more of the radioactive material than the rest of the breast tissue.

Digital Mammography

A magnetic resonance imaging (MRI) machine uses a large magnet and radio waves to measure the electromagnetic signals your body naturally gives off. It makes precise images of the inside of the body, including tissue and fluids. MRI can also be used to see if a silicone breast implant has leaked or ruptured.

PET Scan

Cancer cells grow faster than other cells, so they use up energy faster, too. To measure how fast glucose (the body's fuel) is being utilized, a tracer (radioactive glucose) is injected into the body and scanned with a positron emission tomography (PET) machine. The PET machine detects how fast the glucose is being used. If it is being used up faster in certain places, it may indicate the presence of a cancerous tumor.

Stereotactic Imaging

This special type of mammography machine is used during a biopsy. After mammograms are taken from different angles to locate the exact position of a breast lump, a computer merges the pictures to make a three-dimensional image of the breast. The image is used to precisely guide a biopsy needle to the suspicious area of the breast.

"You gain strength, courage and confidence by every experience in which you really stop to look fear in the face."
Eleanor Roosevelt

Chapter Six
Understanding Breast Cancer and How It Is Diagnosed

Not everything that is faced can be changed, but nothing can be changed until it is faced.
James Baldwin

If an abnormality should appear in one of your breasts, you will want to discover as soon as possible whether it is a benign breast disease or cancer. In order to understand what needs to be done, it is important that you know something about breast cancer itself.

Understanding breast cancer won't enable you to escape the disease, but it could save your life. It saved mine. At present, many things are being studied to prevent breast cancer totally, but for now, early detection remains the key. Remember, if we catch breast cancer in its earliest stage, when it is confined to the breast, optimally we can expect a 95 percent chance of survival. To me, that makes breast cancer worth learning about.

WHAT IS BREAST CANCER?

Every day, cells in your body divide, grow, and die. Most of the time cells divide and grow in an orderly manner. But sometimes cells grow out of control. This uncontrolled growth of cells forms a mass or lump called a tumor. Tumors are either benign or malignant.

Benign Tumors

Benign tumors are not cancerous. But left untreated, some may pose a health risk, so they often are removed. When these tumors are removed, they typically do not reappear. Most importantly, the cells of a benign tumor do not spread to other parts of the body, or invade neighboring tissue.

Malignant Tumors

Malignant tumors are made of abnormal cells. Malignant tumor cells can invade neighboring tissue and spread to other parts of the body. A malignant tumor that develops in the breast is called breast cancer.

HOW DOES BREAST CANCER GROW AND SPREAD?

Just like us, to continue growing, malignant breast tumors need to be fed. They get nourishment by developing new blood vessels in a process called *angiogenesis*. The new blood vessels supply the tumor with nutrients that promote growth. As the malignant breast tumor grows, it can expand into nearby tissue. This process is called *invasion*. Cells can also break away from primary, or main tumors and spread to other parts of the body. The cells spread by traveling through the blood stream and lymphatic system. This process is called *metastasis*. When malignant breast cells appear in a new location, they will begin to divide and grow out of control again as they create another tumor. Even though the new tumor is growing in another part of the body, it is still called breast cancer. The most common locations of breast cancer metastases are the lymph nodes, liver, brain, bones, and lungs.

WHY DOES BREAST CANCER GROW?

We all have genes that control the way our cells divide and grow. When these genes do not work like they should, a genetic error, or mutation, has occurred. Mutations may be inherited or spontaneous. Inherited mutations are ones you were born with—an abnormal gene that one of your parents passed on to you at birth. Spontaneous mutations occur during your life and may have been caused by molecular changes inside the body, or by your exposure to environmental toxins such as radiation or chemicals. But the actual cause or causes of mutations still remain unknown. Researchers have identified some of the genes that are important to cell growth. Errors in these genes turn normal cells into cancerous ones.

But remember, cells may be growing out of control before any symptoms of the disease appear. That is why breast screening to find any early changes is so important. The sooner a problem is identified, the better the chance is for survival.

TYPES OF BREAST CANCER

There are several different types of breast cancer. They are broadly classified into one of two groups: in situ and invasive breast cancer.

In Situ

In situ means that the abnormal cell growth stays within the walls of the ducts or lobules. *In situ* means "in place." Ductal and lobular carcinomas that do not spread outside the duct or lobule are called in situ cancers. They are often called pre-cancerous conditions because they can either develop into or raise the risk of getting invasive cancer. This cancer has not developed the ability to invade normal breast tissue nor to metastasize (travel to other parts of the body).

Invasive

Invasive cancer means that the abnormal growth of cells has spread into nearby tissue. Invasive breast cancer is not the same as metastasis. Metastasis occurs when cancer cells break away from the original tumor and spread to other parts of the body. When ductal or lobular carcinomas spread into nearby tissue, the cancer is called invasive. Breast cancer invades the lymph nodes in about 40 percent of women.

IF AN ABNORMALITY APPEARS

Okay, the worst has happened. You find something abnormal in your breast. What next? Let's go over exactly what should be done, step-by-step, in the event of even the most minute abnormality. I like to use plain language, because I know just how intimidating medical terminology can be. But the more you understand now, the better you will be able to remember the information when you need it most. Keep in mind that no two cases of breast cancer are exactly the same. Diagnosis and treatment procedures must be individualized according to many factors unique to the woman involved. However, it is useful to understand what the options are so that, if nothing else, you have a starting point on which to base your own questions.

"There is nothing to fear except the persistent refusal to find out the truth . . . Fears grows in the darkness; if you think there's a bogeyman around, turn on the light."

Dorothy Thompson

STAGING OF BREAST CANCER

In addition to diagnosing the type of breast cancer a woman may have—in situ or invasive—doctors also look at other growth characteristics such as the size and spread of the tumor. This is done to determine the stage of breast cancer. Three characteristics define each stage:

- ✗ The size of the Tumor of the breast,
- ✗ Whether the cancer has spread to the axillary lymph Nodes, and
- ✗ Signs of Metastasis to other parts of the body.

This is called TNM staging, which ranks the stages of breast cancer from 0 through 4. The earliest and the least serious stage of the disease is 0, with 4 being the most serious stage. Early-stage breast cancer is considered stages 0–2. Which type of treatment your doctor recommends and you choose is based on your stage of breast cancer. Outlined below is a summary of TNM staging.

Stage 0
Tiny cluster of cancer cells in a breast duct or lobule; no spread to the axillary lymph nodes; no metastasis.

Stage 1
Tumor size is up to 2 cm; no spread to the axillary lymph nodes; no metastasis.

Stage 2
Tumor size is smaller than 2 cm; has spread to the axillary lymph nodes; no metastasis present.

Tumor size is between 2 and 5 cm; may or may not be spreading to the axillary lymph nodes; no metastasis.

Tumor is larger than 5 cm; no spread to the axillary lymph nodes; no metastasis.

Stage 3
Tumor is any size; has spread to multiple axillary lymph nodes with the nodes attached to each other or has spread to lymph nodes along breast bone; no metastasis.

Tumor is larger than 5 cm; may or may not have spread to the axillary lymph nodes; no metastasis.

Stage 4
Tumor can be any size; may or may not have spread to the axillary lymph nodes; has spread to other organs of the body or the skin and lymph nodes above the collarbone.

Chapter Seven
Choosing a Support Team

*"A woman is like a teabag. You can't tell how strong
she is until you put her in hot water."*
Nancy Reagan

I f you are diagnosed as having breast cancer, the first
thing you must do is try to stay calm. I realize that
might seem like a silly thing to say. I didn't stay calm, and
I was a well-informed cancer patient. But remember this:
*Being diagnosed with breast cancer does not mean you have
been handed a death sentence.* Anyone who has ever had
cancer remembers what it felt like hearing the diagnosis
for the first time. It is not uncommon to feel angry, afraid,
cheated, depressed, vulnerable and helpless all at the same
time. These emotions are normal, and it's difficult not to
let them overwhelm you. So, before you do anything, get
your mind right. If there was ever a time for a little
self-indulgence, it's now. As Betty Rollin so eloquently
put it in her book, *First, You Cry,* you need to allow yourself to release the emotion you feel after being told you
have a life-threatening disease. Cry, scream, get mad, feel
sorry for yourself—do all of these things if you want. Not
only do you deserve it, but expressing yourself honestly
will help relieve the stress. But as Betty Ford wisely suggested to me, try to limit the hysteria to a short time; then
put it behind you. Carrying on indefinitely will affect your

ability to play the important role you must play in the decision-making process ahead. By acknowledging your emotions and allowing yourself to express them, you can begin to cope, and, in time, learn to take charge of your care and your life as a breast cancer survivor.

Your medical team, family, and friends can help you through the process. In the next several chapters, I am going to try to guide you through this process, as a friend and as a cancer survivor myself. I am not a physician; I wouldn't presume to give medical advice. What I can do for you, what I want to do for you, is to discuss the disease openly and honestly so that you have a basis for actively participating in the decisions about your own care. It's your life, and you need to be in charge.

Women have always been caregivers. My mother is a perfect example. But when it comes to our own care, we have a tendency to put our lives blindly in the hands of physicians. That's certainly what Suzy did. A woman specialist in adult psychological oncology once put it this way: "There is something about seeing the two initials *M.D.* after a name that allows us to give up our right to question their [our physicians'] authority." We must get over this. We owe it to ourselves to ask as many questions as necessary to fully understand our situation and make informed choices. If you don't understand the diagnosis and/or treatment you've been prescribed, you will never be able to fight with the determination and gusto needed to beat this disease.

The best way I know to do that is to learn as much as you can about what your options are and then decide for yourself which ones best serve your needs—psychologically and practically, as well as medically. You need to assemble a team of experts you trust to give you medical advice and emotional support. Then, ask questions, and keep asking until you understand and are satisfied with the answers. You then will be prepared to embark upon the informed decision-making process that will establish your treatment strategy.

With the help of your team of experts, you can take control of the situation. But remember, the final decisions should always be yours.

MY OWN SUPPORT TEAM

My mother always told me never to lose my sense of humor, even in the most difficult situations, because those are the times when it is needed most. Whenever I meet a new physician, whether it is for my own personal health or for the Foundation, I can't help but think of Erma Bombeck's funny quote, "Never go to a doctor whose office plants have died."

When cancer was detected in my left breast in 1984, I affectionately referred to the group of people I depended on most during that crucial time period as my "A Team." But the truth is, this group of individuals was and continues to be a guiding force in my life. None of the people on my team were there by accident. I strategized and thought about each one of them, and they all have their own individual roles in my continued recovery.

The "A" had a double meaning for me: First, it stood for excellence—representing the best possible group of individuals for my own personal needs; and second, it stood for *attack*. After I got control of my emotions, I was determined to attack my cancer with everything I had.

My advantage over some of you is that my team was pretty much in place *before* my cancer was diagnosed. After living through my sister's illness, going through three previous biopsies, and establishing the Komen Foundation, I already knew which individuals would give me the best possible support, both medically and emotionally. I will share with you how and why the members of my team were chosen, though your needs might be completely different. As in all avenues of cancer treatment, what is right for one person is not necessarily right for another. Every case is unique; every woman is an individual. But understanding the way I chose my "A team" might give you a start, if nothing else, in putting together your own. Every cancer patient should have one.

THE FIRST STEP
Finding the Right Physician

If you have a lump in your breast, chances are that it was detected by one of four ways:

(1) You found it through BSE or by accident (which was the way I found my own cancer);
(2) it was noticed by a partner and brought to your attention;
(3) it was discovered by your health care provider during a clinical breast exam; or
(4) it showed up during a screening mammogram.

If the lump was detected by options 3 or 4, your advantage is that at least you are under a physician's care. You have a place to begin, someone to whom you can direct your questions. But if you found the lump yourself or if it was found by a partner, where do you go first? Who do you call?

Ideally, your physician should be someone you trust; someone you feel comfortable talking with; someone willing to answer all your questions. In all likelihood during your treatment and recovery, you will have several physicians; a medical oncologist, a breast surgeon, pathologist, radiation oncologist, and perhaps a reconstructive surgeon. Some programs and centers already have these teams assembled. Because so many specialists are involved in your treatment, however, make sure *you* identify one who will serve as the team leader. This team leader should be aware of all treatments, procedures, medications, and complementary therapy you are receiving.

But what if you are without a physician at all? Perhaps you are new to an area. Usually everyone has access to a nearby hospital that can refer them to a specialist. In the event you are in an underserved part of the country or are not comfortable with the physician you know, there are several organizations listed in the resource section of this book that can help you find a good physician, cancer specialist, hospital, or clinic as nearby as possible.

Take some time to think about what you want in a physician and then schedule a consultation with likely candidates. Everyone has their own wish list when it comes to the "ideal" physician for their needs. There are certain indefinable qualities that make us like one physician over another, and I don't want to diminish the importance of feeling comfortable with whoever you choose. But remember, you're not looking for a new best friend. Although important, there is more to selecting a physician than his or her bedside manner. Think about the characteristics that matter to you in a physician and then take some time to also consider these important physician attributes and qualifications. *Remember, you have some time to decide on your options. You don't have to make final decisions the day of your diagnosis.*

Availability
 ℵ Is she/he a preferred provider on your insurance plan?
 ℵ Does she/he have convenient office hours and
  location?
 ℵ Does she/he spend time with patients?

Qualifications and Experience
 ℵ Is she/he board certified in oncology medicine?

☙ How many years of experience does she/he have treating women with breast cancer?

☙ Has she/he been recommended by a peer physician?

Personal Style

☙ Does she/he take an aggressive approach to treating breast cancer?

☙ Is she/he easy to talk to? Does she/he listen?

☙ Is she/he professional and calm?

☙ Is she willing to let you make your own informed decisions?

THE MEDICAL MEMBERS OF MY TEAM

The most important factor I used in choosing my medical team was trust. I had to trust my physicians completely; I had to believe wholeheartedly that they wanted to see me well as much as I did. Everything I told my physicians was the truth, and I had to believe everything they told me was the truth. No one knows more about your body than you do. Not your partner, your parents, not even your physician. So when you talk with any medical professional about your health, remember that you have valuable information they can use. Share that information. Communication between you and your physician is one of the best ways to make sure you get the care and satisfaction you deserve.

I couldn't have trusted any physician without being aware of his or her work. Knowing your oncologist (cancer specialist) is board-certified (approved by the American Medical Association board in his/her specialty) should provide an element of comfort. To find out whether a physician is board-certified, you can check with the American Medical Association, any of the comprehensive cancer centers, the National Cancer Institute, or the American Society of Clinical Oncology. Or call your county's medical society for a referral. I had the opportunity to interview all my physicians prior to treatment. If you don't have that same advantage, find *one* physician you trust completely and ask for his or her advice.

I also had to like my physicians. This is not to say that I had to become close personal friends with them. If you recall, Suzy needed that kind of relationship with her physicians, and I have always thought that worked to her disadvantage. Having said that, it just so happened that the person I chose to be my head coach, or team leader, was George Blumenschein, my medical oncologist. He was and is a good friend, but that's because we have had the opportunity to develop that kind of relationship over many years. The physicians you choose to make up your team have got to be willing to spend time with you, particularly the person you choose as your team leader.

If George Blumenschein was my head coach, I was the quarterback. I listened to him and the other members of the team and studied their advice, but I insisted on calling the shots. And I was *capable* of calling the shots because I was an educated cancer patient. You can be one, too.

I also had two breast surgeons on my team, Fred Ames and George Peters. I was well aware of Fred Ames's work through the time I spent in Houston at M. D. Anderson with Suzy, although she was not his patient. I had interviewed him several times in conjunction with Foundation projects and knew his work to be first-rate. Fred Ames was the person who performed my mastectomy. George Peters, a breast surgeon in Dallas, where I lived at the time, was always willing to answer any question I might have at any time. He was very helpful to me when I labored with lymphedema, guiding me to find a way to overcome the problem rather than just accepting it. Before making these two men a part of my team, I not only interviewed them, but I also spoke to some of their patients. (If you need help finding a certified breast surgeon, consult the American College of Surgeons or the Society of Surgical Oncology.) Besides the two breast surgeons, I also had two reconstructive surgeons on the team. Being an informed cancer patient, I knew that down the line, reconstructive surgery would be in my best interest, although I wanted to allow enough time to pass to ensure that I had made a good recovery from my initial surgery. Besides the man who actually performed my surgery in Atlanta, John Bostwick, I depended on (and still depend on) a reconstructive surgeon in Dallas by the name of Fritz Barton for wise and sound advice. (Considerations involved in breast reconstruction and choosing a reconstructive surgeon are discussed in chapter 9.)

Another medical member on my "A Team" was Dr. Marc Lippman, a medical oncologist who is now Chief of Internal Medicine at the University of Michigan. I have never been a patient of his, but I greatly respect his mind and the contribution he has made to breast cancer research. Marc has given me a thoughtful answer to every question I have ever asked.

And finally, on the medical side of the team was Dr. Stephen Jones of Charles A. Sammons Center at Baylor University Medical Center in Dallas. Steve has published extensively in the field of clinical research. He has allowed me to impose on him at any time when I've been confused or unsure. He explains things to me in clear language that I can understand—and repeats it, if needed. For this reason, his influence has been immeasurable.

If you think that people of this caliber are unavailable to you, you are mistaken. Ask your primary healthcare physician, your local hospital, or the local medical society. You'll find them ready and willing to help.

I want to say a word or two about insurance coverage—namely health maintenance organizations (HMOs) and preferred provider organizations (PPOs). "Managed care" has changed the environment when it comes to selecting your physician and your healthcare facility. You might not be able to choose your "A Team" as I did. You might be under an HMO or PPO plan. Most physicians are members of some kind of physician network. It is likely that your HMO or PPO will have a wide range of specialists and perfectly good physicians available when you need them.

However, I want you to know that you may have some options under this type of "managed care." If your HMO or PPO does not include the specialist needed to treat you, don't be intimidated. Sit down and negotiate with them to get access to a physician outside the network. Many HMOs or PPOs are willing to do this. And many physicians outside the network will be willing to see you and accept the fee arrangement set by your HMO or PPO.

If you believe you need to get a second opinion from a physician outside your network, check with your insurance to see if this is a covered expense. Remember, most HMOs or PPOs will work with you to provide the best possible care.

Be sure to refer to your insurance coverage booklet or summary of benefits to find out what procedures and treatments are covered under your plan, what your insurance company will pay, and the process for submitting a claim. Get the phone number and name of the claims processor that you can contact when you need assistance in understanding your coverage. Be persistent and patient.

If you are not insured, call Cancer Care for a list of insurance companies that may provide coverage and organizations that may offer financial assistance. Your state insurance commissioner may also be able to give you names of companies that will provide insurance for high-risk or uninsurable clients, or refer you to the Medicaid program.

THE EMOTIONAL SUPPORT MEMBERS

I believe that to have a winning team, a breast cancer patient needs both medical and emotional support. My requirements for the emotional support team were very much the same as for the medical support team. Each member had to have a great deal of integrity and to be honest with me all the time. I needed empathy without sympathy. I needed people who would not allow me to feel sorry for myself, but rather encourage me to continue leading as normal a life as possible. My mother, Ellie Goodman, played a key role in my emotional survival. Without her nurturing every step of the way, I don't know how I would have gotten through the whole ordeal. She never left my side for a moment.

I also received a great deal of strength from talking with other breast cancer survivors. There are many women out there who have given me hope and inspiration without even knowing it. *No one* can fully understand exactly what you are going through unless they have been through it themselves. It is important to seek out positive role models if you are going to get strength from other cancer patients. A positive role model is not necessarily a woman who has beaten the disease, but rather a woman who has never given up her will to live. A positive role model has learned to appreciate life *because* of having breast cancer rather than in *spite of it*. In that way, the late Jill Ireland was and will always be a role model for me, as was my dear friend, the late Nina Hyde, fashion editor of *The Washington Post.* Even when their breast cancer was far advanced, both of these women never gave up or gave in. Another was the late Rose Kushner, a former cancer patient and one of the guiding and leading resources in breast cancer research in this country until her death in January 1990. She not only answered my questions but always left me with a provocative thought to ponder long after our conversation ended. Rose Kushner helped me become a stronger cancer survivor.

Another member of my non-medical team was my good friend, Sharon McCutchin. Besides being an active volunteer for the Komen Foundation, Sharon is the one person I can *always* count on for a good laugh. Even in my darkest, ugliest moments, she had the ability to cut through my turmoil and bring a smile to my face. I call friends who accept us without makeup and without hair "low maintenance friends"—the best kind to have.

The last two members of my emotional support "A Team" were my husband, Norman, and son, Eric. Norman, without ever trying and perhaps never knowing, inspired me to try to look good throughout my illness. I never wanted him to know how sick I felt because I didn't want to scare him. Every day I made a conscious effort to fix my hair (or wig, scarf, or turban) and put on my lipstick. If I wasn't up to getting dressed, I put on something colorful. Doing these little things made me feel better, and if Norman hadn't been around, I might not have made the effort. Eric, my wonderful son, of course, loves me unconditionally. Until he left for college, not an evening went by without his telling me he loved me. I think that is a lot to get from a son. He, above all else, provided me with the reason to get well and get well fast.

> *"One hand cannot applaud alone."*
> Arab proverb

YOUR "A TEAM"

That was my "A Team." Once again, what worked for me might not necessarily work for you. Every one of these people was my partner. Your team should consist of the best possible medical advisors you can find, a few people who love you no matter what you say or do, at least one person who will make you laugh, someone who pushes you to your fullest potential, and someone for whom you will always want to look good. You might also need someone to cook and clean for you (yes, husbands and children can do this), run errands, or be an extra pair of ears at the physician's office. Or, you might need someone to just listen or give you a hug when the going gets tough, and it will. Whatever you need, don't be afraid to ask for help. That's what friends and family are for. Once your team is set, together you can plan your winning strategy.

A WORD ON PHYSICIAN/PATIENT RELATIONSHIPS

Long gone are the days when we, as women, must accept whatever is said to us without question or confrontation, especially where our health is concerned. As I said at the beginning of this chapter, the best thing you can do for yourself is to ask your physician as many questions as you need to ask in order to fully understand what has happened, what is happening, and what will happen to your body. Asking questions will also aid in the evolution of good physician/patient relationships based on mutual understanding and open communication. I know that our ability to make informed decisions has increased dramatically in the last two decades thanks to improved education and access to information. You not only have the right to know the reason for every piece of medical advice you receive, it is now your *responsibility* to know. It is my opinion that as physicians get used to the idea of communicating openly and honestly, they appreciate sharing the burden of the crucial decisions that must be made daily in dealing with cancer patients.

The Questioning Process

In developing a successful relationship with your physician, keep in mind that he or she must be treated with the same respect you insist upon for yourself. While you may be overwhelmed by your diagnosis, it is still necessary and important to get the most out of each physician's visit. Try following these guidelines:

- ❈ *Be prepared.* It is often helpful to gather information about your health concerns from the library (books and medical journals), the Internet, or fact sheets. The more you know, the more comfortable you'll be talking to your physician.
- ❈ *Write down your questions.* Avoid closed-ended questions that will give you a "yes or no" answer. Instead, ask open-ended questions like, "What are the chances of a woman in my situation surviving?" and "What treatment do you recommend?"
- ❈ *Tell your story.* When your physician comes in, ask if you can take a few minutes to briefly explain your situation and concerns. Be as specific as you can. Then give your physician your list of questions.
- ❈ *Give feedback.* If your physician's responses were helpful, say so. This kind of feedback will encourage him or her to talk with you, listen to you, and continue to help you.

Sometimes a woman can be so preoccupied with the fact that she has cancer that it is nearly impossible for her to remember the answers to the questions she has so painstakingly prepared. This is a normal reaction. Don't be embarrassed but be even better prepared next visit. Get a journal and take notes. Or bring a tape recorder to your physician's office so you can play the tape containing both your questions and the answers later, at a time when you feel more relaxed and better able to hold onto the information. Another option might be to bring a relative or close friend to the consultation with whom you can discuss the outcome later to make sure you both registered the same information.

The most important thing is that you *ask* the tough questions no matter how frightened you are of the answers, no matter how uncomfortable it is to discuss a subject as intimate as your breasts with a virtual stranger.

What questions should you ask? I can give you a guideline, a place to begin. You can and should add to this list whatever else you want to know. No question is silly or stupid when you are fighting for your life!

- ☧ What, specifically, did my biopsy show?
- ☧ What surgical procedures are used to treat breast cancer?
- ☧ What are the potential risks and benefits of these procedures?
- ☧ Which procedure and treatment plan are you recommending for me, and why?
- ☧ Where will the surgical scars be located?
- ☧ How can I expect to look and feel after surgery?
- ☧ Why do physicians take lymph nodes from the armpit area?
- ☧ When will you know about my lymph node involvement?
- ☧ What role does lymph node involvement play in my overall health picture?
- ☧ Is there any indication that my cancer has spread?
- ☧ What are the results of my hormone receptor assays? (Your physician might not have the results for seven to fourteen days.) What treatment is indicated by these results? Do I need an HER2 test?
- ☧ What about the aggressiveness of my tumor? How quickly is it growing? What factors helped you to determine this? What does this mean in terms of treatment?
- ☧ What neoadjuvant therapy, if any, would you recommend?
- ☧ Will I need any treatment beyond surgery? Why (or why not)? What supplemental treatments are available?
- ☧ (If non-lumpectomy patient) Am I a candidate for breast reconstruction? If so, what options are available to me?
- ☧ If I am a candidate, what steps should be taken to assure successful reconstruction?

These are just a few of the first things you will probably want to know as soon as breast cancer has been diagnosed. After a specific treatment has been suggested, I'm sure you will have a lot more questions. As we discuss the different treatment options in the next chapter, I will add to that list of questions just as you will.

Speaking in Positives

The first question that comes to every woman's mind when she is told she has breast cancer is *Am I going to die?* For many years, cancer and death were two words that went hand in hand. This is not the case anymore. More people are surviving cancer every day. Breast cancer, detected in its earliest stages, has a high percentage of successful outcomes. Although it is an understandable question, asking if you are going to die is a very difficult question for any physician to answer. It is also very negative and immediately presents an unfavorable state of mind. To put yourself in a more positive state, try to ask questions such as: What can *I* do to beat this? Or what can we do as a *team* to ensure my best chances of survival? You have every reason to feel hopeful about getting through this. If you want more constructive answers, ask more constructive questions.

Still, you need to know the facts. Sugarcoating a situation never cured anyone. Suzy is proof of that, too. No physician is doing you a favor if he glosses over the seriousness of your condition. But wouldn't you rather think that you have an 85-percent chance of survival rather than a 15-percent chance of death? Even if I was told I had a 10-percent chance of survival, *that's* what I would hold on to.

Second Opinions

Once you've prepared your questions, listened to the answers, and discussed them thoroughly, what happens if you are not satisfied with the information you've received? Are you stuck? Let me tell you about my friend Richard Bloch in Kansas City. You might have heard of him, as he is the cofounder of H & R Block, the income tax specialists. In the late 1980s, Richard was diagnosed with what was said to be "terminal and untreatable" lung cancer, caused by many years of smoking. His surgeon told him to go home and get his will and estate together, because there was no hope. Well, that was not the answer he wanted to hear. Richard and his wife, Annette, furiously researched the disease. Because of its reputation and willingness to help him, he checked himself into M. D. Anderson Cancer Center. After undergoing radiation therapy, chemotherapy, surgery, immune system stimulation, and psychotherapy, Richard learned that his condition was indeed treatable. "There is no type of cancer for which there is no treatment, and there is no cancer from which some people have not been cured," he insists.

There is a lesson in Richard Bloch's story for all of us. Asking for a second opinion should never make you feel uncomfortable in any way. Whenever cancer is involved, the situation is serious. Sometimes even a third or fourth opinion is necessary before you feel secure about both the diagnosis and the prescribed treatment. Most physicians welcome the support of their peers. If the opinions differ, the only thing that should matter to any physician is your health. Just think, after literally receiving a death sentence from one physician, Richard Bloch has had many more years of quality life and is still going strong. Doesn't that sound like a great reason to ask for a second opinion? Today, in an effort to reduce the high cost of medical treatment, many insurance companies recommend and pay for a second opinion before agreeing to underwrite any form of treatment at all. Some insurance companies and HMOs actually require you to get a second opinion, and most physicians will not be offended that you want a second opinion

Teamwork

The most important aspect of establishing a successful physician/patient relationship is teamwork. I can't stress it enough. The reason cancer is such a dangerous disease is that it is difficult to control. Knowing exactly what is going on and having a say in your treatment is the only way of getting back some of the control your cancer has taken away. I don't care how brilliant a physician might be, if he or she did not allow me to be a partner in my treatment, I'd find a new one. I think you should, too. On the other hand, you can't be a good partner unless you make an effort to gain as much knowledge as you can from as many sources as possible. Many physicians have gotten into the habit of making all the decisions because *we have allowed them to make all of our decisions.* If you feel your physician is worth keeping, but doesn't know how to make you a partner, *teach him or her.*

Dr. Marc Lippman describes physician/patient relationships this way: "Imagine you are in a department store and the clerk seems anxious to help you, knowing and expecting you to be a motivated buyer. He or she seems willing to walk the aisles with you, explore the drawers and bins for obscure merchandise, or call the warehouse to see if there is anything new on order, which might suit you better. This is the spirit you should expect from your doctor." Genuine concern for your recovery, genuine desire to find the most appropriate form of treatment for your particular case, and genuine likeability—it's not too much to ask.

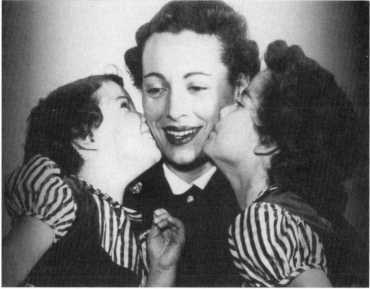

Nancy and Suzy (right) share a kiss with their mother, Ellie Goodman.

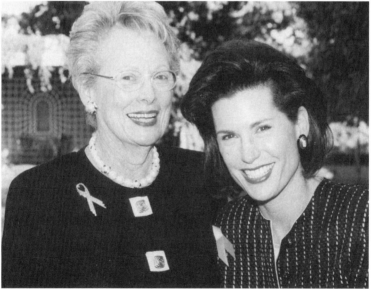

Nancy Brinker and her mother, Ellie Goodman (left), at a reception honoring the Komen Foundation's Million Dollar Council in 1998.

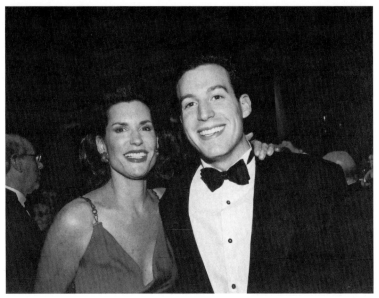

Nancy Brinker enjoys a close relationship with her son, Eric, who resides in New York City.

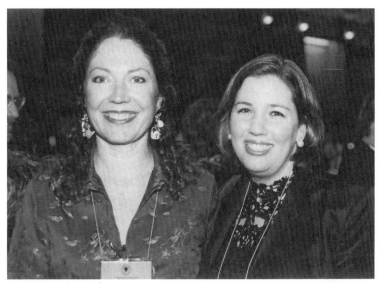

Diana Rowden, former chairman of the Komen Foundation Board of Directors, and Stephanie Komen, daughter of Susan G. Komen, at a recent Komen Affiliate conference.

Scott Komen, son of Susan G. Komen, seen here with his wife, Marnie, and daughter, Susan Madeline Komen.

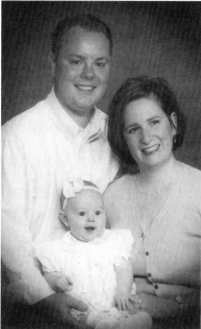

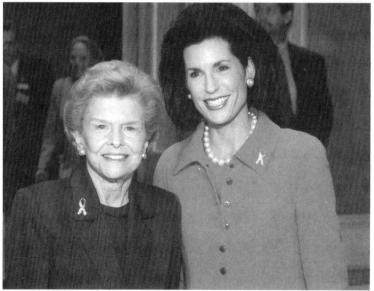

Former First Lady Betty Ford (left) and Nancy Brinker enjoy a long-term friendship and the special bond breast cancer survivors share with each other.

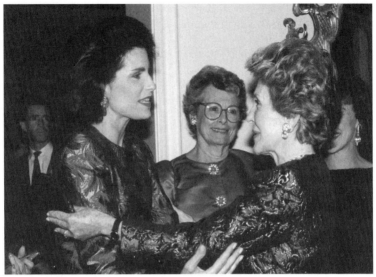

Nancy Brinker (left) and her mother, Ellie Goodman (center), chat with former First Lady Nancy Reagan at a Komen Foundation patron's party held in Dallas. Mrs. Reagan, a breast cancer survivor, is a longtime supporter of the Foundation's mission.

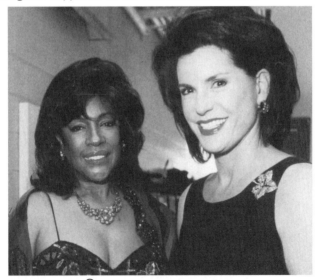

Sing for the Cure,® an original 10-movement choral symphony dedicated to those affected by breast cancer, was held in Dallas in 2000. This musical event featured a beautiful composition, powerful inspiration, and a host of important guests, including Mary Wilson of The Supremes (left), seen here with Nancy Brinker.

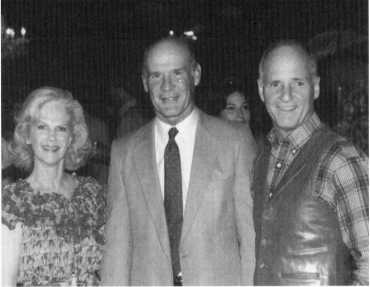

The late legendary Dallas Cowboys football coach Tom Landry (center) and his wife, Alicia, converse with Norman Brinker at a 1986 Komen Foundation event.

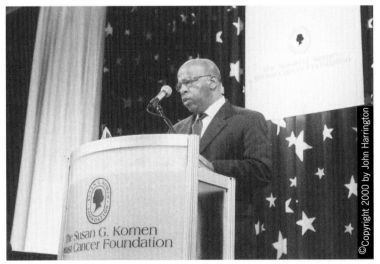

Congressman John Lewis of Georgia was the inaugural recipient of the Champion of Change Award at the 2000 Komen Public Policy Luncheon. Congressman Lewis has demonstrated a remarkable commitment to advancing the interests of minorities and the medically underserved nationwide.

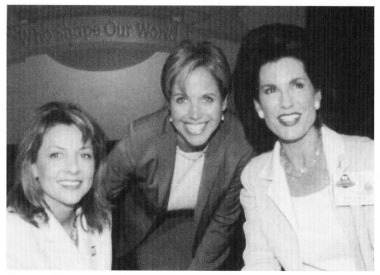

Easter Seals' Beverly Kirby Jones (left) joins famed television personality Katie Couric (center) and Nancy Brinker as they were each honored as "Women Who Shape Our World" in 2000 by L'eggs Hosiery.

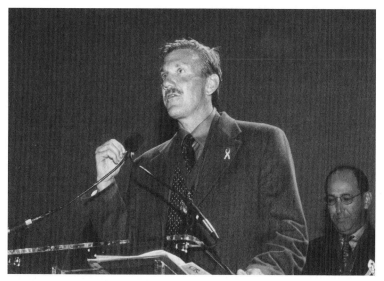

NASCAR racer Dale Jarrett, a friend of the Komen Foundation, has joined Komen's quest to find a cure for breast cancer. When he's not on the race track, Jarrett, the father of two daughters, donates both time and funds to the cause.

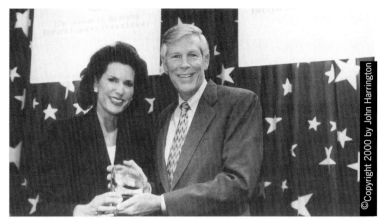

Nancy Brinker presented Senator Connie Mack of Florida with the first annual Komen Lifetime Achievement Award at the 2000 Komen Public Policy Luncheon. Senator Mack, whose wife, Priscilla, is a breast cancer survivor, has demonstrated a devout commitment to cancer causes during his political career.

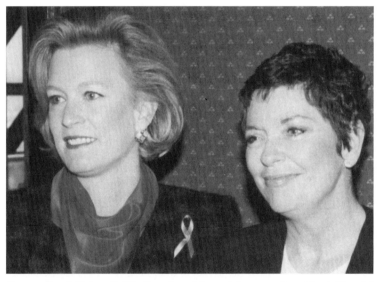

Susan Ford Bales (left), the daughter of former President Gerald Ford, longtime Komen supporter and volunteer (Tulsa and Albuquerque), was on hand in 1993 when the Betty Ford Award was given to television personality, writer, and breast cancer survivor Linda Ellerbee. The honor is named after Ms. Bales's mother, who is a breast cancer survivor and a longtime friend of Komen.

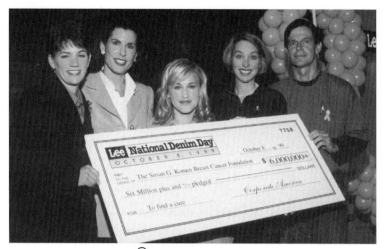

Lee National Denim Day,® the nation's largest single-day fundraiser for breast cancer, benefits the Komen Foundation. On hand for the 1999 check presentation was (from left) Jennifer Lucas, survivor spokesperson; Nancy Brinker; actress Patricia Arquette, celebrity spokesperson; Kathy Collins, vice president of marketing of Lee Company; and Gordon Harton, president of Lee Jeans.

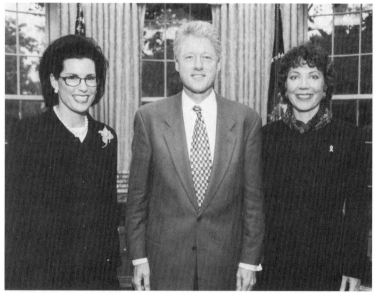

Nancy Brinker and former chairman of the Komen Foundation Board of Directors, Diana Rowden (right), visit with President Bill Clinton during a visit to the White House in the mid-1990s.

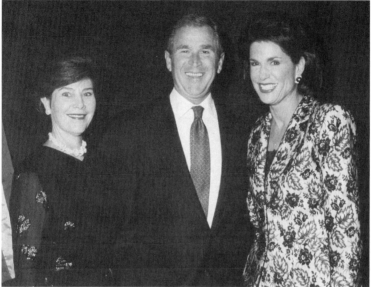

Nancy Brinker joins President George W. Bush and First Lady Laura Bush, who have demonstrated commitment and support for the breast cancer cause and the Komen Foundation over the years.

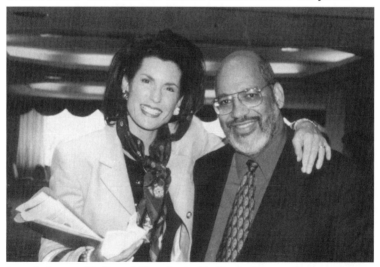

Lovell Jones, Ph.D., of Houston's M. D. Anderson Cancer Center has devoted much of his personal and professional life to studying minorities and cancer. He receives Nancy's congratulations at the 1999 Komen National Awards Luncheon for his efforts as co-chairman of the Intercultural Cancer Council.

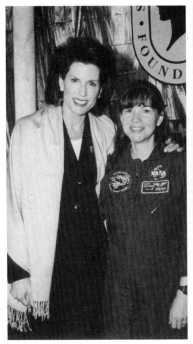

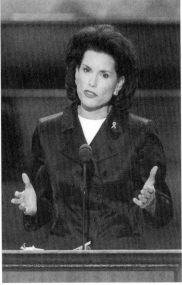

Top right: Nancy addressing a national convention. (Photo copyright 2000 by David Woo.)

Top left: Astronaut Catherine G. "Cady" Coleman gets a hug from Nancy at a recent Komen Affiliates Conference. Ms. Coleman presented Nancy with a pink ribbon that she carried throughout her five-day mission in space aboard Space Shuttle Columbia.

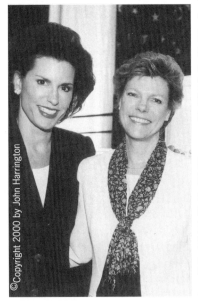

Left: Cokie Roberts, National Public Radio senior news analyst and a noted authority on the U.S. Congress, was emcee at the 2000 Komen Public Policy Luncheon, an important part of the Foundation's annual Mission Conference held in Washington, D.C. She is joined on stage by Nancy Brinker.

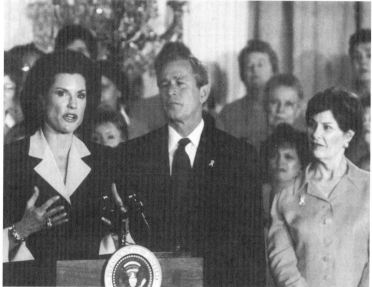

Nancy Brinker speaks to the nearly 300 breast cancer survivors and Komen Foundation supporters who gathered at the White House in June 2001. President George W. Bush and his wife, Laura, as well as Secretary of Health and Human Services Tommy Thompson (not pictured), hosted a breast cancer round-table, followed by a celebratory rally.

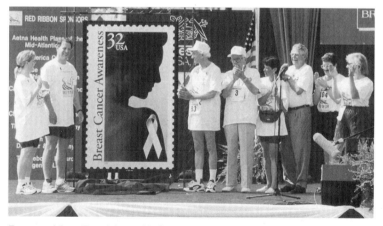

Former Vice President Al Gore and his wife, Tipper, along with former Postmaster General of the United States, Marvin Runyon (third from left) and supporters, witness the unveiling of the first Breast Cancer Awareness Stamp at the Komen National Race for the Cure® in 1996.

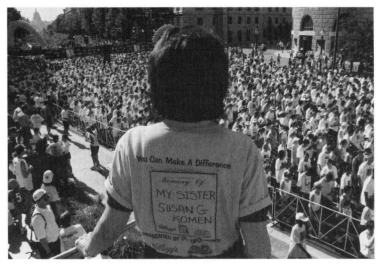

Nancy Brinker, proudly wearing the name of her sister, Susan G. Komen, overlooks the sea of more than 70,000 participants at the 2000 Komen National Race for the Cure.® The Komen National Race for the Cure® is credited as the world's largest 5K fitness run/walk and takes place annually in Washington, D.C.

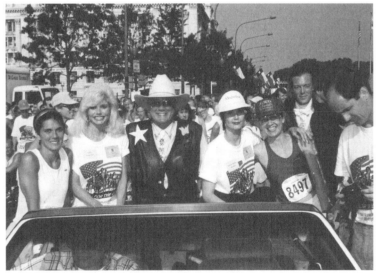

Loni Anderson (second from left), Larry Hagman, and Lynda Carter (second from right) share a moment with two Race participants at the second annual Komen National Race for the Cure® in Washington, D.C., in 1991.

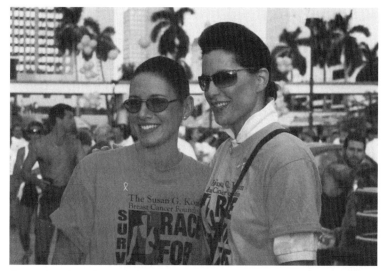

Famed Latina singer/songwriter Soraya (left) shares the sisterhood of survivorship with Nancy Brinker at the 2000 Komen Miami/Ft. Lauderdale Race for the Cure.® Soraya is a gracious friend and supporter of the Komen Foundation.

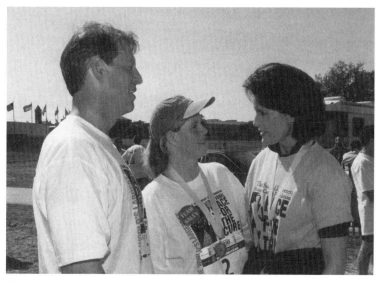

Former Vice President Al Gore and his wife, Tipper, pause to chat with Nancy Brinker at the 2000 Komen National Race for the Cure.® The Gores served as honorary chairs of the Komen National Race every year during their eight-year term in Washington, D.C.

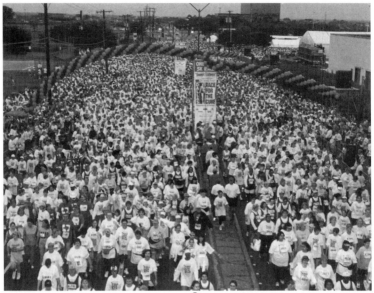

The first Komen Race for the Cure® was held in Dallas, TX, in 1983 with 800 participants. In 1997, 16,300 loyal participants pounded the pavement at the Komen Dallas Race for the Cure.®

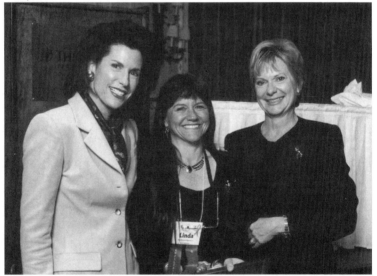

Nancy Brinker (left) and Linda Kay Peterson, Komen Foundation chairman of the board (right) congratulate Dr. Linda Burhansstipanov for her efforts in breast cancer research within Native American populations at the 1999 Komen National Awards Luncheon.

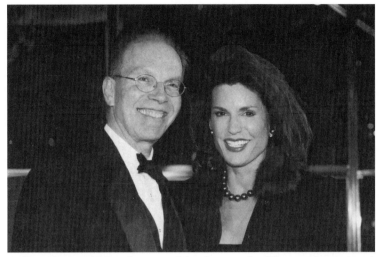

Jeffrey Koplan, M.D., director of the Centers for Disease Control and Prevention, congratulates Nancy Brinker for being among the CDC's Champions of Prevention award winners at a ceremony in January 2000. Nancy was recognized for her pioneering efforts on behalf of breast cancer research, education, screening, and treatment.

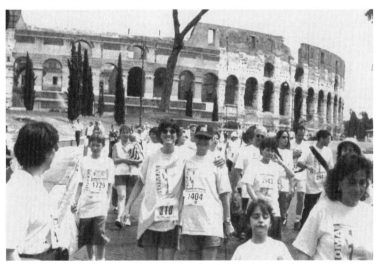

Diane Balma (left), senior counsel and director of public policy at the Komen Foundation, participates with Linda Kay Peterson (right), Komen Foundation chairman of the board, at the Komen Roma Race for the Cure.® The first international Komen Race for the Cure® event was held in Rome, Italy, in 2000.

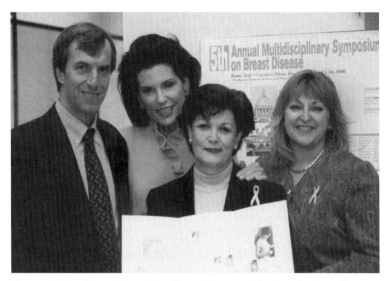

From left: Dr. Riccardo Masetti, president of the Komen Foundation's Italian Affiliate; Nancy Brinker; Dr. Shahla Masood, professor, associate chair of University of Florida Health Science Center, and chief of pathology; and Susan Braun, president and chief executive officer of the Komen Foundation, display two celebrative breast cancer stamps issued in Italy to promote the early detection of breast cancer. The Italian Affiliate was instrumental in having this postal stamp released in an effort to raise awareness of the disease in the community.

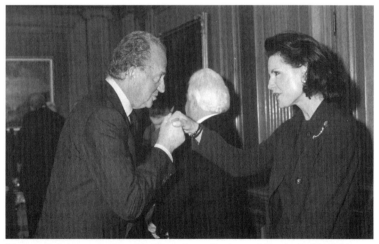

Nancy Brinker meets with King Juan Carlos of Spain in Madrid.

Chapter Eight
Your Treatment Options

"Just go out there and do what you gotta do."
Martina Navratilova

Twenty years ago when I began the Komen Foundation, I could only dream about the kind of treatments and therapies that are available today to women who have been diagnosed with breast cancer. If you've been diagnosed, you have a wide range of options that weren't available to my Aunt Rose or Suzy, or even me, for that matter. I'll admit that not all of them are pleasant; but as Dolly Parton says, "If you want the rainbow, you gotta put up with the rain."

It's up to you to find out what all your options are so you can discuss them intelligently with your physician, your family, and your friends. The treatment plan your physician recommends for you depends upon many factors—the size of your tumor, its type, whether the cancer has spread to lymph nodes or other parts of your body, and your medical history. When your physician suggests a treatment plan, it is important that you understand what guided that recommendation.

Take some time to learn all you can about your type of breast cancer and your treatment options. Try not to let anyone pressure you into making a decision before you are ready. Your breast cancer took a long time to develop, and it is not going to get worse overnight. Days and weeks are fine, months or years are not. You have time to get the information you need to make the right decision. Visit the library, search the Internet, request pamphlets from health care providers and organizations that help cancer patients, and (I can't say this enough) ask your physicians all your questions so you understand your options.

STANDARD TREATMENTS

There are four standard forms of treatment for breast cancer: surgery, radiation therapy, chemotherapy, and hormone therapy. Beyond that, there are other investigational treatments being researched, such as bone marrow transplants. Biologic therapy targets specific cells. Surgery and radiation are local forms of treatment, affecting only the treated area. Chemotherapy and hormone therapy are systemic forms of treatment, affecting cancer cells and noncancerous cells throughout the body by circulating through the bloodstream and the lymphatic system. In order to treat all aspects of the disease, physicians often prescribe a combination of treatments. Usually, surgery is the primary treatment or initial treatment, and the other forms are used as follow-up or adjuvant therapy. However, in some cases chemotherapy might be given prior to surgery to reduce the size of the tumor. This is called neoadjuvant chemotherapy. The course of treatment your physician suggests will depend on several different factors such tumor type, stage, and location, hormone and other receptor status, your age, and your medical history.

Surgery

Surgery is the oldest and most common form of cancer treatment. Although it remains an important part of cancer treatment today, surgery is now typically combined with other types of treatment such as radiation, chemo-

and biologic therapy, and hormone therapy to achieve greater success. There are two main types of surgeries for breast cancer: breast conserving surgery and mastectomy. With breast conserving surgeries, the surgeon tries to spare and preserve as much of the breast tissue as possible, while with a mastectomy the entire breast is removed.

Three types of breast conserving surgeries, which are usually followed up by radiation therapy, include:

- ✗ *Lumpectomy:* A lumpectomy is the procedure in which the surgeon removes the breast cancer and some normal tissue around it, and usually performs a lymph node or sentinal node dissection.
- ✗ *Partial or segmental mastectomy*: In a partial or seg-mental mastectomy the surgeon removes the cancer, some of the breast tissue, and possibly the lining over the chest muscles below the cancer, and usually some lymph nodes under the arm.
- ✗ *Quadrantectomy:* This procedure involves removal of the quarter of the breast containing the tumor plus some skin and the underarm lymph nodes. This sur-gery is usually accompanied by radiation therapy. Like the partial mastectomy, the quadrantectomy might be beneficial to large-breasted women in saving their breast, but for the smaller-breasted women, this pro-cedure may not have a favorable cosmetic result and is often not preferred treatment.

Types of mastectomy include:

- ✗ *A total (or simple) mastectomy*: The surgeon removes the entire breast and usually some lymph nodes or sentinal nodes from the underarm.
- ✗ *Modified radical mastectomy*: The surgeon removes the breast, most of the lower and middle lymph nodes, the lining over the chest muscles, and some-times part of the chest wall muscles.
- ✗ *Radical mastectomy:* Rarely done now, a radical mastec-tomy involves removing the breast, chest muscles, and most of the lower, middle, and upper lymph nodes.

You should discuss any surgical choices thoroughly with your "A Team" and decide together which procedure best fulfills your medical and psychological needs. Naturally, the first question most women have is, *Can my breast be saved?* This is a normal question, an understandable question, but should be secondary to the question, *Can my life be saved?*

The advantage of the lumpectomy is that the breast is saved, often making the disease psychologically easier to handle. In addition to the size, shape and location of the tumor, an important consideration in determining the appropriateness of this type of surgery is the woman's breast size and the amount of tissue to be removed. For example, a small-breasted woman might not have a good cosmetic match to the remaining breast. Other scenarios when a lumpectomy may not be recommended include early stage pregnancy; two or more tumors in more than one quadrant of the breast; a tumor larger than five centimeters; inflammatory carcinoma (an aggressive form of breast cancer); collagen vascular disease (an auto-immune disease that makes it difficult to effectively treat the breast with radiation); and a history of high-dose radiation to the chest or breast. Studies have shown that the majority of women with early-stage disease—Stages 1 and 2—treated by breast-conservation procedures and radiation have the same survival rate as women treated with mastectomy.

Considerations

When determining your surgical, or primary, treatment, two factors are taken into consideration above all others: first, which form of surgery will provide your best chance of recovery, and second, which form of surgery will give you the best possible cosmetic results (appearance). Although modified radical mastectomy is the most common surgery, lumpectomy followed by radiation is being performed more often. For some, the fear of losing a breast can be more traumatic than the fear of cancer itself. This fear is what keeps many women from mammography screening and from practicing breast self-exam. With a lumpectomy, women may take comfort in the knowledge that breast cancer does not necessarily mean the automatic loss of the breast.

However, two women with the exact same size cancerous lesion will not necessarily benefit from the exact same surgery. Remember, I had a very small malignancy in my left breast, but because of its location, a lumpectomy was not my best option. The cosmetic results of a lumpectomy would have been more disfiguring than those of a modified radical mastectomy followed by breast reconstruction. A woman with very small breasts or a tumor located close to the nipple has to think carefully about what procedure will be better for her in the long run. Sometimes even if a lumpectomy is a clinical option, it is not the best cosmetic option.

As you can see, the surgical options you have are quite varied. Which surgery is right for you will become obvious after discussing your test results with your team of physicians.

One note of caution: Something that a lot of women may not know but should consider is that certain types of breast cancer treatments are more common in some regions of the country than in others. For example, mastectomy is more common in the South and the Southwest, while breast conserving therapies are more common in the Northwest, West, and Midwest. This happens because physicians tend to recommend the treatment with which they are most familiar. Be aware of these trends when choosing your treatment.

Radiation

Radiation Therapy (also called radiotherapy) is the use of high-energy rays, usually X rays, to kill cancer cells. Radiation is very effective in killing fast-growing cells like breast cancer. Some healthy cells may also be damaged during radiation therapy, but these can recover. Sometimes radiation is given before surgery to shrink tumor cells. But most often it's given after surgery to stop the growth of any cancer cells that remain. This reduces the chance of the cancer recurring. For example, women who have had a lumpectomy without radiation therapy may have as much as a 40 percent risk of recurrence. This risk is reduced to about 10 percent when radiation is given after lumpectomy.

If you are having radiation therapy, you should not be going through it alone. At this point in your treatment, your expanded medical team should include:

✗ *A radiation oncologist*—a physician trained in using radiation to fight cancer.
✗ *A radiation physicist*—to make sure the machine delivers the right amount of radiation.
✗ *A radiation therapist*—to run the radiation therapy machine.
✗ *A dosimetrist*—to figure out how much radiation is needed.
✗ *A radiation therapy nurse*—to help manage side effects and provide information about the treatment.
✗ Other team members may include a dietitian, physical therapist, or social worker.

Here's what you can expect during radiation therapy:

✗ You will meet with your radiation oncologist to discuss your treatment in detail.
✗ You will have a one- to two-hour planning session called a simulation. A radiation therapist will pinpoint the exact area that will receive radiation (called the

treatment port). Treatment ports will be marked on your skin with indelible ink or semi-permanent tattoos. These marks help the therapist aim the radiation at the same area every time you have treatment. Be careful not to wash these marks off, and tell your therapist if they start fading.

- You will meet with a radiation therapy nurse to discuss skin care, diet, and how to cope with possible side effects.
- Your radiation oncologist, dosimetrist, and radiation physicist will meet to decide how much radiation is needed, how it should be given, and the number of treatments needed.
- Your treatment will begin one or two days after the simulation. Daily treatment time ranges from seconds to several minutes, and is done on an outpatient basis. The typical course of treatment is five days a week for about five to seven weeks.

The room in which the radiation will actually be administered can be a bit intimidating at first. You will lie on a composite, nonmetallic table under a large machine—a linear accelerator—from which the radiation is dispersed. The technician will spend as much time as it takes to ensure that you are in just the right position. It is of the utmost importance that you do not move after you have been correctly positioned because the entire procedure would be useless if the radiation misses the intended tissue. The technician will then leave the room to avoid exposure to the radiation, and you will be observed through a closed-circuit television. The standard dosage administered to the entire breast for early stage breast cancer is somewhere between 4400 and 5000 centigray (one centigray equals one rad). By using small amounts of radiation daily, less damage is caused to normal cells, allowing them to recover more quickly.

Radiation therapy does not hurt, but there are a few common side effects you might or might not experience in the treated area such as:

✗ *Skin irritation* and redness in the treatment area: This side effect is similar to a sunburn, causing the skin to peel, itch, and feel dry. Treat your skin like you would for a sunburn. Not all lotions and sunscreens can be used during treatment so check with your physician first. Cover up when you are outside and use a sunscreen of SPF 15 or greater. Wearing a soft cotton bra without underwires can also help.

✗ Many women are *fatigued* during radiation therapy, so it is important to get rest and to eat nutritiously in order to keep up your strength. Your body is using a lot of energy to heal itself. Try to also get as much sleep as possible. If you can, adjust your work schedule or activities to give you more time to rest.

✗ *Dry cough or difficulty in swallowing.* This is most likely to occur if the lymph nodes in the neck or near the breast bone are also being treated. Eating cold, soft foods like gelatin or ice cream can help ease your throat discomfort.

✗ *Breast changes or swelling.* Your breast may become sore on a long-term basis. You may help alleviate some of the discomfort by wearing loose cotton clothing and not wearing a bra.

Each of these side effects can be inconvenient or uncomfortable, but never fear, they will pass when your treatment is completed.

As is the case with any breast cancer treatment, radiation can fail to stop the recurrence of the cancer, requiring a mastectomy at a later date. However, studies show that most women treated for breast cancer by primary radiation therapy after a lumpectomy are as pleased with the outcome cosmetically as they are with the improved survival rate and prognosis.

Approximately four to six weeks after the first course of treatment, a "boost" dose of radiation is given in the same area of the breast where the tumor was removed. There are two types of boost treatment. The most common one is given externally (as in the first course) and may last from one to two weeks. The other type of boost is called internal radiation therapy where a radioactive substance (an implant) is inserted into the tumor area. Usually the implant remains in the breast two to three days before it is removed. It is, in fact, a precautionary procedure, which attempts to ensure that all the cancer cells have been destroyed.

The implant procedure will require a short hospital stay, probably no more than two or three days, and is done usually under general anesthesia. Thin plastic tubes are threaded through the tissue where the original tumor was taken out. How many tubes are used depends on the size and location of the tumor that was removed. To make sure that the tubes are correctly in place, a chest X ray will be taken. Then you will be taken back to your room, where the radioactive material (iridium) is inserted into the plastic tubes.

During these two or three days, you will receive approximately 2000 rads to the site of the original tumor and surrounding tissue. The procedure is not painful, although you might experience slight discomfort at the time the tubes are being put in place and removed, much like the feeling of stitches being put in and taken out. This discomfort can be minimized with medication.

You will not be confined to your bed but will be able to move around the room freely. It is necessary to stay in a private room because the implant emits small amounts of radiation that might possibly put other people in the room at risk. Visitors must stay at least six feet away, and it is not recommended that children or pregnant women enter the room at all. This is just a precaution, as the amount of radiation received by visitors is not thought to be large enough to be a health risk. After the two or three days, the plastic tubes will be removed and you will be discharged from the hospital.

Considerations

You will probably have a lot of questions about radiation before you can commit to this form of treatment. Just the name alone can be frightening. Here is a list of possible questions you might want to ask during your initial consultation. There are probably other questions you will want to add to the list. Ask as many questions as you need, and keep asking until you have enough information to make an informed decision.

- ℜ Why do I need radiation therapy?
- ℜ After reading my pathology report, viewing the slides, and examining me, do you feel the size, location, and type of tumor I have will be responsive to radiation therapy? Will you explain why (or why not)?
- ℜ How does the radiation work?
- ℜ Are normal tissues damaged in the process?
- ℜ How many treatments will I have and what is the dosage I receive?
- ℜ What is the course time and dosage of radiation therapy?
- ℜ How often will I be seen by a physician during the course of the treatment?
- ℜ What kind of machine will be used? What are its advantages and disadvantages?
- ℜ How reliable is the machine? How often is it unable to function? How old is this machine?
- ℜ Who administers the treatment? If it is a technician, how experienced is he or she? How closely is he or she supervised?
- ℜ How long does each treatment take?

✗ Should I come alone, or should a friend or relative accompany me?

✗ What side effects might occur and how long do they last? Which side effects should be reported to the physician or nurse?

✗ Would any special diet or dietary supplement eliminate or lessen the side effects?

✗ Are follow-up visits with a physician necessary upon completion of therapy? How often are the checkups and tests required after completion?

✗ I understand that ink markings can leave residue on clothing. Can I use tattoos, if I prefer? What does tattooing involve?

✗ What are the precautions or prohibitions during and after treatment (e.g., use of skin creams and lotion, underarm shaving, etc.)?

✗ Is it all right to continue normal activities such as work, sex, and sports during and after treatment?

✗ How soon should treatment begin? What are the risks if I delay or miss a treatment?

✗ Do you recommend other forms of treatment in conjunction with radiation therapy? Why (or why not)?

✗ What is the cost of radiation therapy? Is it usually covered by medical insurance? (Check your own policy's terms.)

Chemotherapy

Chemotherapy is the use of anti-cancer drugs to treat cancer. It can be used to keep cancer from spreading, slow the growth of cancer, or kill cancer cells that have spread to other parts of the body. Chemotherapy is given after surgery (called adjuvant chemotherapy) or before surgery (known as neoadjuvant therapy) to reduce the risk of recurrence. Since chemotherapy is a systemic treatment—the drugs circulate in the body through the lymphatic system and the bloodstream—unlike surgery and radiation, it can reach tiny cancer cells called "metastases." While some of these metastases might be detected by X rays, CT scans, bone scans, or physical examination, often (particularly in the early stages) they might be undetectable by currently available tests. For this reason, chemotherapy is invaluable as a weapon against cancer. Today, adjuvant therapy (given in addition to surgery and radiotherapy) is used earlier in cancer treatment in addition to surgery and radiation in the attempt to prevent or postpone a cancer recurrence. Chemotherapy has also been successfully used to shrink large breast tumors that have not spread to other parts of the body, which allows a woman more surgical options.

Chemotherapy can be administered orally through pills or into a vein (IV) through the arm or through a specialized type of venous access catheter. There are several types of these and you should discuss them with your physician.

Like every other form of cancer treatment, however, chemotherapy has its own set of disadvantages. Because it cannot, as of yet, distinguish between fast-growing cancer cells and fast-growing "normal" cells in the body, there are many potential side effects associated with chemotherapy. The most obvious are loss of hair, loss of energy, nausea, vomiting, a cessation of your menstrual period (this is sometimes permanent), anemia, and susceptibility to infection. There are others, as well, which might or might not occur depending on your particular prescription and dosage, such as deterioration of bone marrow, mouth ulcers, rashes, changes in skin pigment, blood in the urine caused by bladder inflammation, lung damage, and weakness of the heart. And like any treatment, there is always the possibility that chemotherapy will not work in much the same way one builds up a resistance to other drugs.

Experiments and studies are being done every day to improve the effectiveness of chemotherapy while diminishing its side effects. There is also a great effort being made to simplify chemotherapy so that women on chemotherapy can continue with their regular lifestyles as much as possible.

Types of Chemotherapeutic Drugs

There are many different drugs used in a variety of combinations being used today to treat all kinds of cancer. The good news is that many of these drugs are effective in treating breast cancer. Let's go over each of them so that when you and your oncologist discuss them, they won't seem completely foreign.

> ☧ *Alkylators* work by damaging genetic material that controls tumor cell growth. An example is cyclophosphamide (brand name Cytoxan).
>
> ☧ *Antimicrotubule agents* work by preventing cancer cell division. Examples include: paclitaxel (Taxol), docetaxel (Taxotere), and vinorelbine (Navelbine).
>
> ☧ *Antimetabolites* work by interfering with the cancer cells' ability to produce RNA and DNA and are especially effective in killing dividing cells. Examples of antimetabolites effective in treating breast cancer are 5-Fluorouracil (5-FU) and methotrexate.
>
> ☧ *Antitumor antibiotics* have a completely different meaning when used in the treatment of cancer than when used in the treatment of infections, because in this case, the antibiotics destroy tumor cells, not bacteria. Doxorubicin (brand name Adriamycin) and Epirubicin, aka anthrocyclines, have proven particularly effective in treating breast cancer.

These are just a few of the most common drugs you are likely to hear about when discussing chemotherapy; you might hear about others. New drugs are being developed and tested every day. Try not to be alarmed by the sound of their names. Remember, scientists and physicians have a language of their own. Each drug has its specific purpose, and you have a right to know exactly what is going into your body and why. If you don't understand what a term means, don't be embarrassed to ask. It's also important to know that chemotherapy is usually given as combinations of drugs. Several common combinations include "FAC" or "CAF" (5-FU + Adriamycin + cyclophosphamide), "AC" (Adriamycin + cylophosphamide), sometimes followed by paclitaxel (Taxol) "CMF" (cyclophosphamide + metho-trexate + 5-FU). These combinations use several drugs to attack the cancer cells simultaneously and are usually more effective than one drug alone.

Considerations

Many women are afraid of having chemotherapy because of its side effects and the toll it can take on the body. Although chemotherapy does have a dramatic effect on the body, it is often a successful treatment. It reduces the risk of cancer returning after surgery and can kill cancer cells that have begun to spread to other parts of the body. And physicians know more about chemotherapy than ever before. The doses are more accurate, and there are a variety of medications to help minimize side effects.

But expect some changes in your life during chemo-therapy. Your daily routine will be affected. You may be able to continue to work and keep doing your normal activ-ities. Or you may be too tired to do all the things you nor-mally do. That's okay. Your friends and family can help. You will start to feel better once the treatment is over. Until then, listen to your physician or nurses who can give you suggestions on how to manage your daily activities.

Factors such as your tumor's stage, hormone recep-tor status, rate of breast cancer cell division, lymph node involvement, as well as your age, menopause status, other medical conditions, family, social, and job factors, will all enter into your decision. You should participate in the decision with your physicians to decide whether chemotherapy is right for you.

Physicians, nurses, and pharmacists have become very skilled at giving chemotherapy in ways to minimize side effects, while maintaining cancer-fighting capabilities. For example, considerable care goes into the determination of individual doses of drugs by the pharmacist. The doses are carefully calculated based on your height and weight and are adjusted if side effects occur. The blood counts are carefully monitored, and growth factors to stimulate blood cell production may be used also. Anti-nausea agents (antiemetics) are available to reduce or eliminate the vomiting and nausea that can occur with chemotherapy. Eating several small meals throughout the day and not drinking liquids during meals can also help.

I still remember how much I hated losing my hair. But then I think of the alternative. I wish there were a way to eliminate hair loss, but right now losing your hair is still a frequent side effect to chemotherapy. Your hair may get thinner or may fall out completely, depending on which chemotherapy drugs you are given. Your hair will grow back after treatment is over. Using mild shampoos, soft hairbrushes, and low heat when drying your hair can help reduce hair loss. If you would like to wear a wig, it is a good idea to get it before treatment begins if you want to match your hair color and style.

Some other possible side effects of chemotherapy include infections (since your white blood cell count is now lower) and mouth and throat sores (because the fast-growing cells of the mouth are killed). Although the reason is unclear, some women also experience weight gain during chemotherapy. Also, loss of menstrual periods and menopausal symptoms like hot flashes, irritability, or difficulty in sleeping may occur. Your health care provider can help minimize these side effects.

The side effects of chemotherapy are almost always temporary, but occasionally they aren't. It is a risk every cancer patient must face. I personally think the risk is worth taking.

However, you have to make your own choices. Sometimes the quality of life, even in shorter time increments, is more important than the quantity. What constitutes life quality and changes is very individual and also depends on the stage of a particular cancer, the age of the patient, and the patient's lifestyle. What was right for me might not be right for you. We all have to respect the individual choices made by each cancer patient. I just want to make sure that every woman with breast cancer understands the seriousness of the disease and is aware of all the options open to her. Breast cancer is a formidable opponent. To win the war, *you have to fight.*

Here is a list of common questions most often asked when chemotherapy is prescribed. Use it as a guideline and add to it whatever you need in order to have a better understanding of your treatment.

- ✗ What, specifically, is chemotherapy, and why is it indicated in my case?
- ✗ What is the significance of lymph node involvement in relation to chemotherapy?
- ✗ How many of my nodes are involved or affected by the cancer?
- ✗ What were the results of my hormone receptor assays, biomarker tests, and how quickly is my breast cancer growing? What other tests did you run? How did the results of these tests influence your treatment suggestions?
- ✗ Which chemotherapy drugs are you recommending for me? Why have you chosen those particular drugs rather than another combination?
- ✗ How long will I need this treatment?
- ✗ How frequent are the treatments?

✗ How are the drugs administered?

✗ How long does each treatment take?

✗ Should I come alone for the treatments, or should a friend or relative accompany me?

✗ Tell me all the possible side effects I might experience. Are they permanent? Does everyone get them?

✗ Is there anything I can do to lessen or relieve the side effects?

✗ How much do these treatments cost? Will they be covered by my health insurance?

Chemotherapy has proven its effectiveness in making many cancer patients cancer free for the rest of their lives. Other times, it doesn't work at all; still for others it can add a few good years to their lives. To me, knowing all the risks, enduring this often unpleasant form of treatment was worth every minute of suffering I experienced, though at times during the treatment it didn't always seem that way. You must think about all the benefits, weigh them against the negatives, and decide for yourself what is best for you.

Hormone Therapy

Like chemotherapy, hormone therapy is a cytotoxic, systemic treatment that kills cancer cells directly. Hormones are substances naturally produced by the endocrine glands. Their purpose is to stimulate other organs. Hormones are largely responsible for reproductive functions such as ovulation and milk production and for aspects of appearance that distinguish the genders. When cancer begins in tissues that are affected by hormones, such as the breasts, it is possible the tumor will be affected by hormones as well. You may also hear some physicians call this approach "anti-hormone therapy" since the purpose is to prevent hormones from attaching to these cancer cells and stimulating their growth.

Originally, hormone therapy as a treatment for breast cancer was limited to the surgical removal of hormone-producing glands, as in an oophorectomy (the removal of the ovaries). Today, however, while surgery to remove the ovaries might be desirable in treating cases where the production of hormones by the body is believed to be speeding up tumor growth, synthetic drugs such as tamoxifen, toremifene, megestrol acetate, anastrozole, and goserelin have been proven to control recurrent breast cancer and produce long remissions from the disease as well. Once again, the names of the drugs are more intimidating than the drugs themselves. The truth is that in many cases where hormone therapy is an option, the side effects are much less severe than with chemotherapy. In rare cases, however hormone therapy might cause serious side effects such as depression, blood clots, or rarely, endometrial (lining of the uterus) cancer.

Estrogen and progesterone are naturally-occurring female hormones that some breast cancers need to grow. Tumors that have many sites to which these hormones attach are known as hormone receptor positive. A receptor-positive tumor often needs hormones to grow. If a woman has estrogen or progesterone receptor-positive breast cancer, she has a tumor that may need estrogen or progesterone to grow.

The drug tamoxifen has been shown to be an effective treatment for both early and advanced stage breast cancer. It is widely used for women who have had breast cancer in one breast to reduce the chances of cancer developing in the opposite breast, and as a preventive therapy for women who are at high risk for breast cancer. Tamoxifen is given in a pill form and works by blocking estrogen from binding to estrogen receptors in estrogen receptor positive breast cancers. Anti-estrogens and aromatase inhibitors are effective treatments for estrogen and/or progesterone positive breast cancers.

For women with estrogen receptor-positive breast cancer, taking tamoxifen for five years significantly reduces the risk of recurrence of a breast cancer and the risk of dying from breast cancer. For women without a personal history of breast cancer, tamoxifen can reduce a high-risk woman's chance of getting breast cancer in the first place by 50 percent. Tamoxifen may also decrease the risk of osteoporosis (bone loss) and heart disease. Common side effects may include hot flashes, vaginal dryness, and vaginal discharge. These are similar symptoms commonly experienced by women during menopause. A few women may experience mild nausea, weight gain, fatigue, or depression. One rare but potentially serious side effect is an increased risk of developing a blood clot in the lungs (pulmonary embolism) or in the major veins in the legs (deep vein thrombosis which occurs in only 1 percent of women). Because about 1 percent of women taking tamoxifen may develop endometrial (uterine) cancer, routine gynecological exams are recommended. Let your physician know if you are having any of these problems.

It is crucial that a hormone receptor assay be done at the time of the biopsy to determine whether or not hormone therapy is an option for you, and that you be made aware of the results. The presence of estrogen and/or progesterone receptors in the breast cancer is thought to be associated with higher survival rates and long-term remissions. However, if your hormone receptor assay proves to be negative, as mine was, you can still achieve optimal results through chemotherapy and/or radiation in conjunction with your initial breast surgery. Clearly, the best advantage of having a positive hormone receptor assay is that it gives you another option in treatment.

Considerations

Here are some questions you might want to know the answers to before considering hormone therapy. As always, use them along with your own questions.

- ✗ What is hormone therapy?
- ✗ Was my breast cancer estrogen receptor (ER) or progesterone receptor (PR) positive? If so, what does this mean?
- ✗ Which hormone drugs are you recommending for me, and why?
- ✗ In what form will the treatment be given, and how often will treatment be given?
- ✗ How long will I be on this treatment?
- ✗ Should I have hormone therapy in conjunction with any other forms of treatment?
- ✗ What if hormone therapy does not work for me? What other choices do I have?
- ✗ What are the side effects I might encounter, and what, if anything, can I do to prevent them from occurring?
- ✗ What is the cost of hormone therapy and will it be covered by my insurance?

NEW APPROACHES TO TREATMENT

Now that we have discussed the standard cancer treatments, let's talk a little bit about newer treatments that are not as proven at this time: biological therapies, bone marrow or stem cell transplantation, clinical trials, and alternative and complementary therapies.

Biological Therapy: The New Frontier

I refer to biological therapy as the new frontier in breast cancer research because it is such an exciting field of research and offers real hope for the future. Scientists are now beginning to understand cancer at its most basic cellular level. This means they are getting closer to discovering what causes a normal cell to change into a cancer cell. To me this sounds like a great breakthrough. I can't help but wonder, however, what will happen thirty years from now if, in a moment of rare nostalgia, my son Eric should pick up this book with his own son or daughter and glance through the pages. Do you suppose they'll laugh at what I once thought was a great breakthrough? Maybe. One promising biological therapy agent is the drug trastuzumab (Herceptin). In certain women with metastatic breast cancer, Herceptin has been shown to shrink tumors and slow the spread of cancer. A clinical trial in women with metastatic breast cancer has shown Herceptin's benefits when combined with chemotherapy or when used alone.

Immunotherapy

Under normal circumstances, the body's immune system recognizes a foreign invader, seeks it out, and attacks it. When a bacteria invades your body, for example, the body responds by producing antibodies to help fight off the bacteria. But the body does not effectively recognize cancer cells as foreign invaders. Immunotherapy helps by activating the body's immune system to recognize and attack cancer cells. One type of immunotherapy being evaluated in clinical trials is cancer vaccines. Cancer vaccines seek to stimulate the immune system so that it can more effectively kill cancer cells.

Perhaps the greatest hope for the treatment of breast cancer in the future will come from therapies that are based on an improved understanding of the way in which breast cancer begins and progresses. Dr. Marc Lippman offers us the simple yet useful analogy of asking a cave man to try to stop a car's engine. If he takes out a club, there is no question that sooner or later he could get the car to stop, but by then the car would be reduced to a complete wreck. While this might be an overstated analogy for chemotherapy and radiation treatment, it is also clear that these therapies can damage normal as well as abnormal parts of the body. A more rational understanding of how a car works leads to half a dozen strategies which could conceivably stop the car without damaging it, such as turning off the ignition, siphoning out the gas, pulling off the distributor cap, etc. In the same sense, as we start to understand the specific components that set a cancer cell apart from normal cells (its ability to grow continuously in an unregulated fashion, its ability to invade structures and tissues, and finally, its ability to break away from the parent tumor mass and spread throughout the body), we will be able to design therapies that "shut it off."

Gene Therapy

A gene that provides sensitivity to a specific cancer-treating drug is transferred to a patient's cancer cells, making the cells more susceptible to the drug. This susceptibility will allow the drug to be more effective in killing the cancer cells. Early gene therapy clinical trials are underway for advanced breast cancer.

Scientists have identified two specific genes thus far that are important in the development of breast cancer. They are called BRCA1 and BRCA2. Every woman has these genes, but some women have inherited a mutated form of one or both genes. Inheriting a mutated form of BRCA1 and BRCA2 increases a woman's risk of breast and ovarian cancer. But not all cases of breast cancer are due to inherited mutations based on what we know to date. Inherited gene mutations, including mutations to BRCA1 and BRCA2, account for only 5 to 10 percent of all cases of breast cancer, while most breast cancers are due to some kind of spontaneous gene mutations.

The likelihood that you have mutations in the BRCA1 or BRCA2 genes is greater if one or more of the following statements are true for you:

❧ Your mother, sister, or daughter has had breast or ovarian cancer
❧ A woman in your family has had both breast and ovarian cancer
❧ A woman in your family has had pre-menopausal breast cancer
❧ A woman in your family has had breast cancer in both breasts
❧ Your family is of Ashkenazi Jewish decent

But remember, most women who get breast cancer do not have an inherited gene mutation on BRCA1 or BRCA2. That is why it is important that you perform monthly breast self-exams and have clinical breast exams and mammograms as needed.

You can find out if you have an inherited gene mutation by being tested. Ask your physician for a referral to a genetic counselor. These counselors are trained health professionals who can interpret a woman's family history of breast and ovarian cancer as well as the results of the genetic testing. The steps a woman can expect to go through include:

STEP 1: You will undergo a thorough evaluation of your family history and explanation of your individual risk.
STEP 2: If you decide to proceed with genetic testing, you will attend pre-test counseling. This counseling includes:

❧ An overview of the genetic testing procedure
❧ A review of the risks and benefits of gene testing, such as cost, confidentiality, and the potential knowledge that you carry the gene mutation

✘ A discussion of what you will do with the information once you know the test result

✘ A discussion of the emotional impact of this
information, as well as implications for your
family.

STEP 3: A sample of your blood will be drawn for the
test.

STEP 4: The sample will be sent off for testing. It usually takes four to six weeks to obtain results.

STEP 5: Interpretation of the results will be explained to
you by the genetic counselor.

The Komen Foundation has funded genetic research in
the laboratory as well in a clinical setting. Dr. Mary
Claire King of the University of California at Berkeley
was a Komen research grant recipient. Her genetic
research discoveries have been of major significance in
unlocking critical genetic information in the progression
of breast cancer.

If you are interested in genetic testing, you should talk
to your physician who can refer you to a genetic counselor
in your area. Or you may contact the National Society of
Genetic Counselors (found in the resource section of this
book) for a referral to a health center near you.

Bone Marrow or Stem Cell Transplantation

Bone marrow, or stem cells, are collected from your
body, stored, and then returned to your body following
high-dose chemotherapy. Bone marrow and stem cells
are important in the blood forming system of your body.
By removing them prior to chemotherapy, they are not
damaged by the chemotherapy agents, and can help your
body recover after the chemotherapy is given. Although
proven effective in some cancers, bone marrow/stem cell
transplant for some stages of breast cancer is still being
studied in clinical trials. Research is now underway

comparing high-dose chemotherapy with bone marrow transplantation to standard chemotherapy to see whether or not bone marrow transplantation is more beneficial than standard therapy in breast cancer.

Clinical Trials and Research Studies

Clinical trials and research studies involving patients with breast cancer are important sources of information on new treatments. Clinical trials are often the only way to translate theoretical research progress into real cancer therapies; and for many patients, they offer the best treatment available. Many of the breakthrough therapies saving the lives of women with breast cancer today are the direct result of clinical trials conducted in years past by hundreds of dedicated researchers working with thousands of women determined to beat their cancer.

Unfortunately, only 3 to 4 percent of all adult cancer patients participate in clinical trials that might save not only their own lives but also millions of others stricken with breast cancer in the future. It is essential that these valuable studies get the public and private support needed to continue this crucial research so that medical science can move closer to finding a cure.

I was lucky. I was placed in a clinical trial that has proven to be very successful. If I had to make a choice about whether or not to participate in a clinical trial again, I would do it in a heartbeat. Some women feel that being a part of a study group makes them a "guinea pig" for scientists; I disagree. Today, cancer treatment has become so advanced that you will always be given some form of studied treatment which will be compared against another form of proven standard treatment to see if there is a slight or marked advantage for one or the other.

You can find out what clinical trials are being done, and where, by contacting PDQ (Physicians Data

Query), a computerized information service that provides physicians and patients with the most up-to-date cancer information possible. PDQ can tell you who has the state-of-the-art facilities and where the newest tests are being conducted (see the resource section). When you call or visit the PDQ website, you will need to know your diagnosis, including type and stage of cancer, where the primary cancer is located, cell type, and address and phone number of the physician who is providing your treatment (see the resource section or log on at www.nci.nih.gov).

The NSABP

For many years a wonderfully dedicated man, and my good friend, Dr. Bernard Fisher, headed the National Surgical Adjuvant Breast and Bowel Project. The NSABP is one of the nation's oldest and largest ongoing cancer clinical trials networks. It is sponsored by the National Cancer Institute and involves thousands of physicians at hundreds of sites in the United States and Canada.

Beginning in 1958, the NSABP brought together a group of surgical oncologists to investigate adjuvant therapy for breast and bowel cancer. Adjuvant therapy is treatment such as radiation or chemotherapy used as a supplement to the primary form of treatment, which is surgery. This group pioneered the now well-established breast-conserving procedure of "lumpectomy followed by radiation" as an alternative to mastectomy.

Through the years of study, the NSABP has concluded that there is equivalent survival for the procedure of "lumpectomy followed by radiation," as compared to mastectomy. Lumpectomy followed by radiation allows breast cancer patients to keep their breast. According to the American College of Radiology and the American Cancer Society, at least one-third, and perhaps as many as one-half, of all breast cancer patients could have a choice in how their cancer is treated. Breast cancer patients should talk with their physician about treatment options in order to make informed decisions.

In 1992, the NSABP began a large Breast Cancer Prevention Trial (BCPT) to study the anti-estrogen drug tamoxifen as a preventative agent for breast cancer in women who are healthy but at high risk of breast cancer. This trial showed that tamoxifen is preventing breast cancer in some high-risk women. Because of the pioneering work of Dr. Fisher and his colleagues, these and other studies done by other cooperative groups offer more treatment for breast cancer patients and greatly improve the quality of life for breast cancer survivors.

Complementary and Alternative Therapies

Rose Kushner once said, "Remember, today's quackery may be tomorrow's breakthrough!" She was referring to the fact that scientists might be open-minded but need to prove theories with hard research and testing. Complementary or alternative therapies can be controversial but are becoming more common in the treatment of a wide range of diseases including breast cancer. The National Institutes of Health now has an office dedicated to the study of complementary and alternative medicine (CAM), and according to the *Healthcare Forum Journal*, between one-third and one-half of all medical schools now offer courses in alternative, complementary, or integrative medicine.

Complementary medicine research is also a part of the Komen Foundation's research portfolio. Let me give you a couple of examples. With the help of a Komen grant, Dr. Anna Wu of the University of Southern California is exploring the role soy may play in the lower incidences of breast cancer we see in Asian women. In a slightly different look at the Asian diet, Dr. Jane Teas of the University of Massachusetts Medical Center is conducting the first experimental study to examine how dietary seaweed and soy either together or independently, might alter hormone levels to help us fight breast cancer.

Some people might think seaweed research sounds a little strange, and I suppose it does. But remember, once upon a time, people thought it "strange" and certainly unnecessary to even wash your hands before surgery. Other critics paint alternative and complementary therapies as last-ditch acts of desperation. They're not. In fact, many people are using such therapies already and do not know it. Did you know that prayer, meditation, laughter, and support groups are complementary therapies? So are imagery (imagining your body fighting the cancer and healing itself), aromatherapy (using fragrances to help you feel calm, relaxed or energized) and art therapy (expressing your feelings through art). The healing touch uses human touch to promote healing and help to control pain. This includes massage and chiropractic medicine, acupuncture (using needles to stimulate certain points on the body), reflexology (using touch to stimulate certain points on your feet), and therapeutic touch (rebalancing the body's energy fields through touch).

Dietary change and dietary supplements such as vitamins, minerals, and herbs are being studied as ways to both prevent and treat breast cancer.

Non-traditional forms of healing often represent not only a different way of thinking about disease, but also of thinking about life. These therapies include ayurveda (an Indian system that brings the body into harmony with its environment) and traditional Chinese medicine, which stresses the importance of balancing energy forces.

I investigated this subject with a number of physicians and some of my associates when I served on the

National Cancer Institute's National Cancer Advisory
Board. Just about every physician I spoke to admitted
that most of their patients "do something" in addition to
conventional medicine. Researchers at the M. D. Anderson Cancer Center found that the use of complemen-
tary/alternative medicine is high—83 percent. Another
study found that breast cancer patients are far more
likely to use complementary methods than patients with
other forms of cancer.

The M. D. Anderson study also discovered that
nearly two-thirds of patients did not discuss these alternative therapies with their physicians. This is one of the
most troubling aspects of the complementary medicine
debate and another good reason for more research, but it
is not the only concern. When people attempt to *replace*
conventional therapies with alternative approaches, they
are putting themselves at unnecessary risk.

Although proper diet, the right vitamins, certainly
natural herbs, and exercise are clearly helpful in keeping
the body clean and healthy, so far, none of them have
been proven to successfully stop or even slow down cancer. The isolated cases you might hear or read about are
not, I believe, something to pin your hopes on. One to
two percent of all cancer patients go into what is called
spontaneous remission, cancer remission without the aid
of medicine. When this happens—and it is rare—the situation is the exception, not the rule. Please don't be
fooled into thinking a crazy diet or a mysterious herb is
going to cure your cancer.

A woman I know who has been a good friend for a
long time developed a small breast cancer and was successfully treated and reconstructed. A beautiful, energetic
woman, she seemed to handle her illness with a great attitude and recovered quite quickly. She was a role model to
other cancer patients. Speaking to women's groups about

her experience, she helped many women. A year and a half later, my friend was diagnosed with a kind of lymph node cancer called lymphoma. Her physician advised her to undergo chemotherapy, feeling her chances for a possible long-term remission were excellent. What happened between her recovery from the breast cancer and her development of lymphoma, I'm not sure, but now she wanted no part of chemotherapy or any conventional medicine. She opted for a strict macrobiotic diet as her sole treatment. Afraid that she would be criticized by her friends and physicians, this woman checked into a rather well-known "cancer clinic" across the border. Well, her disease did not regress; instead, it had spread throughout her body. My friend died shortly thereafter.

Perhaps none of us really knows how the treatment for breast cancer affected her. Maybe her side effects were worse than she ever let on. My friend had no children and had been through a painful divorce so her support team was limited. I feel that because she was an educated cancer patient, she simply opted for the quality of life rather than the quantity and knew in her heart what the outcome would be. I really don't believe she actually thought this diet would take the place of medical science. Still, it was her choice to make, and we all must respect her decision whether we agree with it or not. I'm just sad because I loved my friend.

On the other hand, I am in full agreement with trying anything and everything to make the unpleasant experience more tolerable as long as your physicians are aware of what you are doing, and it does not interfere with the primary and adjuvant cancer treatments. During my course of chemotherapy, I found "imagery" particularly helpful. I tried to look at "the big picture" first, thinking that these few months of sickness would be minuscule compared to the rest of the healthy life I intended to live.

At times when it got really bad and I felt so sick, I thought back to childbirth. *That* was much worse. Before each treatment session, I would plan a fun outing for a few days afterward. It didn't have to be anything fancy—a movie with Eric or a quiet dinner out would do just fine. When I started to feel bad, I would visualize myself already there, and I would feel better right away.

I also surrounded myself with a lot of "white light," meaning a lot of positive energy. I tried to be with only people I knew cared deeply for me and for whom I cared deeply. I read poetry and listened to music. When I felt up to it, I took long walks in the sunshine and rode horses. I tried to meditate and made it a point to be thankful for my blessings. Above all, I never discounted the power of laughter or the power of prayer. Spiritual and religious awakening is a subject that is exciting. If you are interested, there are wonderful books describing how to enter a state of personal fulfillment or spiritual peace. I highly recommend them. You can find them in the metaphysical studies or new age section of a bookstore.

I also integrated an alternative vitamin therapy into my own cancer treatment with the knowledge and supervision of my "A Team." When I took highly concentrated doses of vitamins along with a traditional course of breast cancer treatment, it certainly wasn't a commonly accepted approach. It still isn't. Certain antioxidants such as high doses of vitamin E and C, for example, may possibly diminish the effectiveness of chemotherapy, and so it is important to talk to your physician about the vitamin therapy you are taking.

I have to be honest, I don't know what impact, if any, the vitamin therapy had on my recovery. And that's the point. We don't know enough, and because we also don't have a cure for breast cancer, I'm not willing to summarily dismiss any reasonable, safe therapy that could be a breakthrough in the prevention, control or cure of cancer or in the quality of life for cancer patients.

But that doesn't mean I think that all non-traditional therapies have the potential for dramatic change. As a member of the President's National Cancer Advisory Board, I had the distinct privilege of meeting some of the most respected scientists in the country. I have sat in on numerous panel discussions and have witnessed first hand the genuine thrill that is felt when a breakthrough is made. I have also been around when what was thought to be a promising discovery fails in some way—everyone mourns. There is no hidden cure for cancer. When the cure *is* found, the whole world will know about it.

When it comes to complementary research, my own view is simple. My treatment and my personal experiences with other breast cancer survivors have shown me that non-traditional complementary therapies have real potential, but all hypotheses must be tested and proven in the same strict format as is used in any other practical study. The health and safety of all people depend on it.

The important thing to know about any and all forms of cancer treatment is that *you have choices*—no matter how far your cancer has progressed.

Surgery, radiation therapy, chemotherapy, and hormone therapy are constantly being tested and retested for ways of improving the process, and promising and exciting news ways of treating breast cancer are continually being studied. Research your disease. Talk to your A Team. Talk to patients. Call the Susan G. Komen Breast Cancer Foundation National Toll- Free Breast Cancer Care Helpline at 1 800 I'M AWARE® (1-800-462-9273) or visit the Komen Foundation's award winning website at www.breastcancerinfo.com.

Take charge of your care and your life!

Chapter Nine
Breast Reconstruction

*"I don't think of all the misery. I think of the beauty
that remains."*
Anne Frank

After you have a mastectomy, you might decide
that you do not want any more surgery done on
your chest. There are some women who choose never to
have reconstruction following mastectomy. Going
through surgery and/or radiation and chemotherapy
might be all the trauma they want their bodies to endure.
Other women feel that they cannot get along without it.
Knowing that reconstruction can bring back her feminine silhouette might be the determining factor in a
woman's decision to go through with the mastectomy.

Betty Ford laughs when she says that she always
planned to have reconstructive surgery, but every time
she was ready, her husband was off campaigning. For
Betty, reconstructive surgery was not a high priority; for
other women like me, it was very important. Clearly, the
decision to have reconstructive breast surgery is a personal one and depends on several factors including age,
general physical health, and self-image. Having had
breast reconstruction two years after my surgery, I feel
the best thing about reconstruction is its ability to promote a sense of wellness. Although I was successful in

TAKING CHARGE OF BREAST CANCER

getting back to a normal life, it wasn't until after my reconstruction that I could truly begin to put the disease behind me. On one level, the fact that I have had breast cancer will never be completely forgotten. In the back of my mind, there is always a thought of recurrence—that's the negative. However, because my own life was threatened, I will forever appreciate the fact that I am alive and healthy—that's the positive. But now, even though talking about breast cancer has become my career, there are some days that go by in which I honestly forget to include myself as someone who has had the disease. That never happened before I had the reconstruction.

If you are considering this surgery for yourself, you need to know what it entails. There are two major types of reconstructive surgery: *immediate*—at the time of mastectomy—and *delayed*—performed months or years after the mastectomy. Talk to your surgeon about it before your mastectomy, if possible, because you might find yourself a candidate for immediate reconstruction, or if not, the position of the mastectomy incision might affect the later reconstruction procedure.

If you have already had a mastectomy and are just now considering the option of reconstruction, don't worry. Almost every breast cancer patient is a candidate for reconstruction. Scarred, radiation-damaged, grafted, thin, or tight skin, and even the absence of chest muscles do not prevent reconstruction.

"It is the mind that makes the body."
Sojourner Truth

Talking to other women who have gone through the surgery will help you get a new perspective if you are unsure about the procedure. Try to find women of approximately your own age to talk with, as their questions and thoughts might be similar to yours. If you can't find anyone, call the American Cancer Society's "Reach to Recovery" program (see the resource section).

Here are a few things to consider when making a choice:

❧ Are you comfortable with the way your chest looks after surgery? If so, you may not want reconstructive surgery. You may be exhausted and choose to forgo reconstructive surgery for the time being. You can have reconstruction at the time of your mastectomy or wait to have reconstruction at a later time. Discuss your decision with your partner and social support network. You don't have to make a decision right away. Talk with other women who have had reconstruction or have chosen to use prostheses.

❧ If you do not want to do anything permanent, but want to maintain a balanced look when you are dressed, a prosthesis may be more appropriate for you. Prosthesis options are discussed in greater detail in chapter 10.

❧ Are you willing to go through a second surgery? Do you have any concerns about reconstruction procedures?

CHOOSING A RECONSTRUCTIVE SURGEON

The most important factor in choosing a reconstructive surgeon is finding someone who is experienced and technically and medically competent. It is also important to find a sensitive physician who understands the psychological impact breast surgery of any kind has on a woman. Your oncologist and/or surgeon might be helpful in giving you some names of reconstructive surgeons to interview. Or consult the American Society of Plastic and Reconstructive Surgeons (see the resource section).

When talking with the surgeon, discuss your feelings about the procedure openly and candidly. This will help you decide if you are comfortable talking to him or her and able to establish the necessary rapport. Ask to see photographs of the surgeon's work and get the names and phone numbers of some of his or her other patients.

Here is a list of questions that might help you get started in your interviewing process. You will probably have many more to add to this list. As always, you should continue to ask questions until the procedure is clear in your mind.

- ✗ What type of reconstructive surgery do you recommend for me, and why?
- ✗ What are the pros and cons of breast implants?
- ✗ What are the risks and benefits associated with this type of surgery?
- ✗ How much experience have you had with this type of surgery?
- ✗ May I see photographs of other patients who have had the various types of reconstruction?
- ✗ May I speak with other patients about the procedure?
- ✗ What can I expect my reconstructed breast to look and feel like after surgery? How, if at all, will this change in six months or a year?
- ✗ How long will I be in the hospital?
- ✗ How long is the recovery period following surgery?
- ✗ What should I do or avoid doing to ensure a safe and fast recovery?
- ✗ How soon can I have this operation?
- ✗ What else should I consider before committing to reconstructive surgery?
- ✗ What about my other breast?
- ✗ How much will it cost? Will this operation be covered by my insurance?

WHEN SHOULD RECONSTRUCTION BE PERFORMED?

The trend in recent years has been toward immediate reconstruction. Several influences have made this possible. Skin-sparing mastectomy procedures have become more common and this additional available tissue facilitates more predictable cosmetic results. As reconstruction becomes accepted as a routine part of treatment, it is more efficient for the patient to start it at the time of the mastectomy.

To determine what is appropriate for you, I suggest you discuss all the variables with your oncologist, your breast surgeon, and the reconstructive surgeon you have chosen. Together, you should be able to come up with a plan that fits both your personal needs and your medical needs.

TYPES OF RECONSTRUCTIVE SURGERY

There are two common procedures used in breast reconstruction. As in all types of breast cancer treatment, each woman's case is individual and the procedure that is best for you should be discussed thoroughly before a final decision is made.

Tissue Expansion and Implants

This technique is used to stretch the skin to make room for a permanent implant. A small, balloon-like bag is inserted under the chest wall. It is expanded by adding saline regularly until the breast area is expanded to the desired size. The expander is removed and a more permanent saline or silicone gel-filled implant is inserted. The implant is most appropriate for women who do not want a flap procedure and involves the least amount of surgery.

Flap Procedures

In these procedures, your own tissue is used to recreate a breast. These surgeries take the longest to complete and are associated with a somewhat higher risk of a complication. However, because they use your own skin, muscle and fat, the reconstructed breast will more closely reflect your bodily changes like gaining or losing weight and aging. There are three types of flap procedures:

❡ The TRAM flap (Transverse Rectus Abdominous Muscle) is the most common reconstructive choice. Tissue is taken from your abdomen and slid up a tunnel under the skin to your breast area.

❡ *The latissimus dorsi procedure* takes tissue from the shoulder area of your back. This, too, is taken in a tunnel under the skin to the breast area.

❡ *The free flap reconstruction* is the most complicated flap procedure. Tissue is taken from the buttocks or the rectus abdominous muscle and transplanted to the breast area.

Nipple Reconstruction

If desired, nipple and areola reconstruction can be performed after having any type of reconstructive surgery. This procedure is usually done at least two months after the breast reconstruction to allow for correct positioning of the nipple.

For some women, breast reconstruction has a profoundly positive psychological impact. For other women, it is an unnecessary and additional surgery that requires general anesthesia. The decision is one that requires a lot of research and discussion. Whether you choose one of these procedures or not, it is important that you know they exist. A major part of being a strong, assertive cancer patient is understanding all of your options.

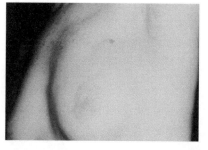

Lumpectomy and under-arm lymph node removal, the most common form of breast preservation.
(PHOTO COURTESY OF DR. GEORGE PETERS)

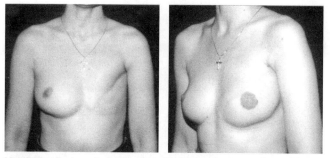

Modified radical mastectomy, currently the most common form of breast cancer surgery, followed by breast reconstruction with tissue expansion.
(PHOTOS COURTESY OF AMERICAN SOCIETY OF PLASTIC SURGEONS)

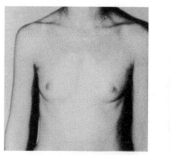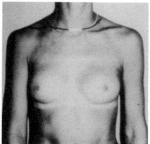

Patient before and after mastectomy and immediate reconstruction with implants.
(PHOTOS COURTESY OF DR. JOHN BOSTWICK)

TAKING CHARGE OF BREAST CANCER

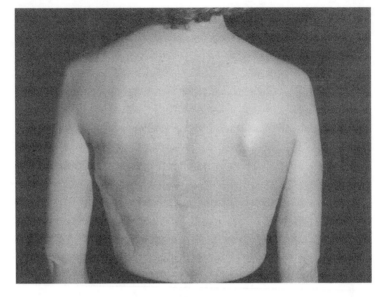

Patient with Latissimus Dorsi scar.
(PHOTO COURTESY OF DR. FRITZ BARTON)

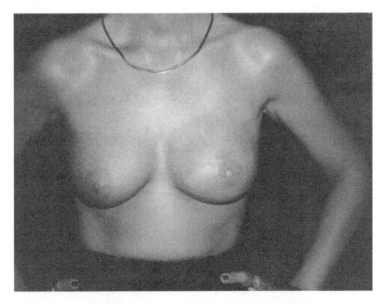

Patient one year later after Latissimus Dorsi
reconstruction and nipple reconstruction.
(PHOTO COURTESY OF DR. FRITZ BARTON)

Chapter Ten
Appearance and Recovery

*"Sex appeal is 50 percent what you've got and
50 percent what people think you've got."*
Sophia Loren

There is probably no other time in a woman's life when she feels less like making herself look attractive than while she is being treated for cancer, yet I know of no other time when the effort is more rewarding.

Believe me, I know first-hand that when you look good, you feel better. I have several friends who lived that maxim. Each was in the depths of cancer despair, but no one would ever have known it to look at them. Mary Tullie Critcher, a former board member of the Komen Foundation and a cancer patient, is one of those women. I distinctly remember her coming to a meeting immediately following a chemotherapy treatment. Most women in her condition would not have shown up for the meeting at all. But Mary Tullie was there, looking more beautiful than ever. She was wearing a soft, silky scarf on her head over which she wore a wonderful hat that matched her dress. The look was quite chic.

Another very special woman was the late GiGi Hill. GiGi was given less than a 5 percent chance of living five years after being diagnosed with metastatic breast cancer in 1980. Knowing exactly what the odds were, GiGi made up her mind that she was going to live those five years to their fullest. In October 1985, GiGi was given the Betty Ford Award at the Komen National Awards Luncheon. She marched up on that stage in front of some fifteen hundred people, shook former First Lady Betty Ford's hand, and flashed her most gorgeous smile. The audience went wild. No one could have guessed from her appearance that she was only days away from death.

HAIR

The most traumatic aesthetic side effect of cancer treatment is, for many, the loss of hair (alopecia). For some women, going out in public without hair is not an option. Other women wear their baldness as a personal sign of dignity and courage. It's strictly up to you.

Scars from surgery can be concealed without anyone knowing about them. Covering a bald head, if that's what you chose to do, may be more difficult. I found the wigs that look the most natural to be the most time-consuming and difficult to put on. Wearing the obviously fake hair was hassle-free, but I had to realize that strangers would know I was sick. It didn't matter—I wanted to get on with my life. The good news is hair loss due to chemotherapy is usually temporary. Also, not all women lose their hair. You may want to have your hair cut short before chemotherapy treatment, to help make the transition to a new style less obvious. In the meantime, try to anticipate what you would do in the event of significant hair loss. You may choose to hide your hair loss by wearing wigs, scarves, false eyelashes and hats or you may decide not to! Use the time before treatment to experiment with different styles and/or colors.

Wigs

In choosing a wig for yourself, try to go to a person or wig salon specializing in the needs of chemotherapy patients.

This is a very emotional and vulnerable time for any woman, and the last thing you need is an insensitive sales-clerk pushing a product that is simply not you. Make sure that wherever you go has a place you can be helped in private. Sometimes an owner will open the salon at "off" hours to ensure your privacy, or if you are really lucky, you may find someone who will come to your home.

Shop for your wig *before* beginning chemotherapy. The salesperson can see your hair color, your particular style, and you can try on different styles to see which one you like best. You might want to take a friend along when you go, or your hairdresser if that is possible.

Wig salons today sell excellent synthetic wigs that look and feel like real hair, but are easier to manage and are a fraction of the cost of natural wigs. Natural wigs are expensive and more difficult to manage. Depending upon the length you choose, an excellent synthetic wig should start at approximately one hundred fifty dollars to two hundred dollars. The synthetic is permanently "set" and you can wash it yourself and style it with a comb and brush. But remember, since your wig is synthetic, avoid extreme heat such as steam, curling irons, or blow dryers. Your wig salon will give you a pamphlet with complete care and setting instructions.

I cut my hair short before I started with the chemotherapy so the change would not seem as drastic to me. Many women find it easier to make the adjustment from short hair to no hair, rather than from long hair to no hair. Some salons suggest that cutting long hair prior to hair loss reduces the weight pulling at the hair, making hair loss less noticeable.

It is difficult to get a true fit for a wig until you have lost all your hair. But get your "new hair" process organized and ready before that time. If you choose a wig before you've lost your hair, ask if you can leave a deposit and pay for the wig later, when you are sure the fit will be correct. If you opt to wait until you can ensure the perfect fit, bring with you a couple of photographs with your hair looking just the way you like it. That way the specialist can do his or her best to make you look as close as possible to the way you are used to seeing yourself.

The concern of every woman who purchases a wig, regardless of the reason, is that it will stay in place. There are several products on the market to ease your anxiety. Wig caps are made of nylon stocking material and help hold the wig in place. Wig liners are made of cotton and serve the same purpose, but can be used as sleeping caps. The cotton sleeping cap is a wonderful idea, for without the protection of hair, your head will get quite cold.

In addition to the wig caps, you may purchase a wig band that has a strip of Velcro® sewn onto it. The wig is placed over the band and adheres to the Velcro.® You can also purchase a two-sided adhesive product that helps hold your wig in place. This product is similar to those used by men who wear hairpieces. However, if you choose to use these strips, you should take extra care when removing the adhesive piece. You may risk skin irritation or infection.

When selecting a wig color, some salons may suggest you opt for one as close to your own hair color as possible. But you may want to have fun and try a new look! If you ever wanted to be a platinum blonde or redhead, this may be the time! After your initial wig purchase, you may want to consider buying a second wig, if that is financially possible for you. That way, while you are washing, drying and styling your original wig, you will have an extra to wear.

Although at this point in your life you are purchasing a wig out of necessity, remember that most of the wigs sold are to women who have hair. Wigs today are quite versatile and very fashionable. Try to make this experience as fun as possible and experiment with different looks. And remember, it is only temporary.

A Note about Insurance

Although every insurance company has its own rules and regulations about what is and what isn't covered, most consider the loss of hair as they would the loss of a limb requiring a prosthesis. Have your physician write out a prescription for a "wig prosthesis" and make sure your wig salon uses the word *prosthesis* on the sales receipt so that it is not confused with a wig purchased for cosmetic reasons. Check the *Yellow Pages* of your phone directory under "wigs," taking care to choose one that specializes in serving the medical patient. If you are unable to afford a wig, contact Y-ME, an organization that maintains a wig bank for women with financial need, or the American Cancer Society's "Reach to Recovery," which may be able to help. See the reference section at the end of this book for contact information.

Scarves and Hats

Scarves are a terrific alternative to wigs. They are fast, simple, and stylish. You can purchase scarves in a variety of different textures and colors to complement any outfit. They should be cotton rather than silk or polyester, as these materials have a tendency to slip around on the head. The best size to use is either twenty-six-inch or a twenty-eight-inch square. There are dozens of different ways to tie scarves into interesting head-wraps, ranging from conservative to a very avant-garde look. Most any department store or accessory store will have books on how to tie scarves. Take advantage of them. The important thing is to develop a style you are comfortable with. Many times, the look is so fabulous, women keep right on wearing scarves long after their hair returns.

Hats can be an equally charming touch to complete an outfit. Berets and caps give you a sporty, fun look; fedoras a more classic, conservative look; and wide-brimmed hats will protect your skin, which will be extra-sensitive at this time, from the sun and wind.

Turbans are a very fashionable alternative to the scarf or hat. A consultant at a shop specializing in wig needs for medical patients gave me a great piece of advice. She said to invest in a "bang" hairpiece to wear under a turban or scarf. That way, if you have put on your makeup, added some jewelry and the bangs, a turban or scarf will look quite natural.

SKIN

Any authority on beauty will tell you repeatedly that even the strongest, thickest skin should be treated delicately. Skin that is being subjected to radiation and/or chemotherapy can be especially tender and sensitive. Be gentle. When washing your face, use a liquid or cream cleanser; they are less harsh than soap. Even if your skin is oily, it is still extra-vulnerable right now. Look for an oil-free cleanser and then follow up with an astringent or whatever your regular routine involves.

Some women find that while going through radiation and/or chemotherapy, their skin is dry, red, irritated, or a combination of any of these, even when normally it is on the oilier side. Moisturizers, skin lotions, and body oils will take away the dry, irritated, chapped feeling caused by your treatments. Occasionally, the skin will react to the fragrance in some of these products. If this should happen to you, don't despair—you will not have to give them up. Almost every major cosmetic company makes a line of products that is fragrance-free. If you are going through radiation, there might be certain restrictions to what you might apply to the area being irradiated, so consult your physician.

Because your skin is sensitive, take your baths and showers in water that is warm rather than hot, especially if you are receiving radiation or have undergone breast reconstruction. After reconstruction, the breast area is numb and has no feeling. Be especially careful to avoid hot water.

If you are experiencing hair loss from chemotherapy, be sure not to neglect your scalp just because there might be little or no hair on your head. If you suffered with the problems of dryness, itching, and dandruff before your hair loss, you will suffer with them during and after your hair loss as well. It is thought that a daily massaging will stimulate blood flow in the area and might produce a stronger, healthier, and shinier head of hair after chemotherapy.

Sun

By now we have all heard about the damage too much sun can do to the skin. Despite the warnings of skin cancer and premature aging, however, some women still spend countless hours in the sun during the summer and never miss a day in the tanning salon during the winter.

It is especially important while you are undergoing cancer treatment to be careful of sun exposure. Too much sun while taking certain chemotherapy drugs can cause permanent changes in the skin pigment.

Still, having a "healthy glow" will be the first you, your family, and your friends will look for as proof that you are well on your way to recovery. Using a sunscreen SPF (sun protection factor) 15 or higher will help keep you safe from the sun's harmful rays (remember to reapply faithfully every two hours and after swimming) and still allow a slow tan. If you want to look healthy but refuse to submit your skin to potential sun damage, don't forget the wonders of makeup. You might also want to try the self-tanning creams that are available. However, check the label to see if they contain sunscreen. If they do not, you will need to apply sunscreen if you are going to be in the sun for an extended period of time. Follow the guidelines of the American Cancer Society by avoiding the sun during its most harmful hours (11:00 AM to 3:00 PM) and wearing protective clothing.

You should also be aware that radiated skin will always be extra-sensitive to the sun. So please take the proper precautions. If you are in any doubt about your personal exposure to the sun or the use of any cosmetic products, always consult your physician.

MAKEUP

Carefully applied makeup can be very helpful at this time. For some women, experimenting with cosmetics is fun, and trying to make yourself look healthy at this time presents an interesting challenge. Even if you have always detested wearing cosmetics, you might want to give them a try. Maybe you've thought the look was unnatural or perhaps you've never wanted to take the time and trouble. You are not alone. Some women prefer a more natural look and feel to their skin. But now, while you are experiencing some of the side effects of breast cancer treatment, you may opt to wear makeup during treatment. You might be experiencing puffiness and either complete or partial loss of eyebrows and eyelashes. A little bit of knowledge on just the basics of makeup artistry can give you the lift you need. Most of the aesthetic side effects of chemotherapy and radiation can be corrected with cosmetics. The American Cancer Society's "Look Good, Feel Better Program" (located in the resource section of this book) provides makeup consultations at no cost.

DRESSING

The two most common treatments for women with breast cancer that affect clothing are the mastectomy and the insertion of a port-a-cath catheter in the vein under your collarbone. Also, of course, there is a short time after a lumpectomy and/or biopsy that you might feel a little sore or uncomfortable, but that should pass within a week or two.

Today, you can dress very casually and comfortably and still be stylish and fashionable. Even with dressier clothes, more attention is paid to comfort now than ever before.

When dressing immediately after surgery or to cover a venous access device, try to wear shirts that are loose-fitting. The catheter sits below the clavicle (collarbone) and halfway between the neck and shoulder. Big, soft collars will cover the area without causing any discomfort. A shirt hides the port-a-cath. Shoulder pads lift the fabric away from the body, keeping the area free from abrasion.

BREAST PROSTHESES

If you have had a mastectomy, you may want to wear a breast prosthesis, which is an artificial device replacing your breast. A prosthesis is an artificial, pliable breast form that you can put on or take off whenever you want. Prostheses come in many shapes, sizes, materials, and colors. A member of your health care "A Team" can suggest nearby places where you can buy prostheses. Many specialty stores that sell medical supplies carry them, as do some larger department stores that have staff who specialize in working with women who have had mastectomies. Before you go, call ahead for an appointment so you do not have to wait. Wear a form-fitting top. Wear the prosthesis around the store for thirty minutes or more to get the feel of it. Try on different ready-made prostheses and decide which one is the best match for your remaining breast. If you have had a double mastectomy, you may buy two matching prostheses. You can also have a prosthesis custom-made. These are more expensive than the ready-made version, but sometimes provide a much better match. Find out what your insurance will cover. Most plans will pay for a reasonably priced new prosthesis every two years. Today, breast prostheses have been revamped for the active woman. They can be worn doing almost anything, even swimming. And, they can be worn with just about any type of outfit except, of course, one that shows cleavage.

Get the "okay" from your physician before being fitted for your prosthesis. The physician will want to make sure the scar has healed and all swelling has gone down. You might want to use one of the soft, unweighted Dacron® breast forms until you can be fitted for a permanent prosthesis.

At night, many women wear a sleep form to bed because the back, neck, and shoulders are susceptible to the same strain lying down as they are standing up and moving around. The sleep forms are not as heavy as the silicone forms worn during the day. They are usually made of polyester, cotton, or foam.

Many women who choose to wear a prosthesis feel just as comfortable with their decision as those who have reconstructive surgery. If you are undecided, you can wear a prosthesis for a period of time. Your emotional recovery walks hand in hand with your personal self-image. Your comfort plays a large role in how you feel and the speediness of your ability to get back into the mainstream. For this reason, when you are fitted for your prosthesis, seek the advice of a qualified expert. Look in the *Yellow Pages* under "artificial breasts" or "prosthetic appliances," or contact the local chapter of the American Cancer Society's "Reach to Recovery" program. The Y-ME organization maintains a prosthesis bank for women with financial need. See the resource section of this book for contact information for these organizations.

LYMPHEDEMA

Lymphedema is a build-up of lymphatic fluid, which causes swelling in the arm and hand, and occasionally in the chest/breast on the side of the surgery. When the lymphatic system is damaged, fluid collects in the tissue of the affected area causing swelling. The surgical removal of the lymph nodes in the underarm area and/or radiation therapy to the affected area can interfere with normal lymph drainage.

The lymph system consists of lymph vessels, nodes, and tissue. Its role is to remove impurities from the body's tissue and to produce cells that are vital in fighting infections. Lymph vessels transport colorless fluid (lymph) that passes through the nodes, where fluid is filtered.

Some warning signs that you may have lymphedema include:

✗ A heavy feeling in your arm
✗ Tight sensation in your arm or hand
✗ Swelling in your arm or hand
✗ Decreased flexibility in your hand or wrist
✗ Shirt sleeves or jewelry that feels tight
✗ Skin that may "pit" with any finger pressure

Let your physician know immediately if your affected arm or hand is warm, red, or swollen, or if you have a fever. These symptoms could indicate an infection and may require an antibiotic.

Here are some good ways to reduce your risk of developing lymphedema:

✗ Have injections or blood drawn from the unaffected arm.
✗ Have your blood pressure taken from the unaffected arm.
✗ Wear gloves when doing housework or yard work.
✗ Keep your arm clean and dry. Moisturize your skin after bathing.

✗ Protect your skin from the sun with sunscreen (at least an SPF 15) and protective clothing.

✗ Avoid lifting or carrying heavy bags, purses, or other objects with your at-risk arm.

✗ Avoid wearing tight jewelry or clothing.

✗ Avoid cutting your cuticles during manicures.

✗ Use an electric razor, not a blade, to shave your underarm.

✗ Use insect repellent when outdoors, but wash it off when inside.

✗ Avoid any type of injury, including scratches and bruises, to the at-risk arm.

✗ Rest your arm in an elevated position (above your heart or shoulder) to help increase the flow of lymphatic fluid. When flying in an airplane, wear a compression sleeve and drink lots of fluids during flights.

✗ Use a compression sleeve. This device is an elastic, custom-fitted sleeve that applies pressure to help fluid drain. It can be used alone or with manual lymphatic drainage.

✗ Employ manual lymphatic drainage. This procedure consists of a gentle arm massage to stimulate movement of lymphatic fluid. It is done by a trained, certified therapist.

✗ Do mild exercise. Staying active will also increase the flow of lymph fluid. Arm stretches will help you maintain range of motion. Activities like swimming and walking will help with circulation. Avoid strenuous and repetitive exercises, and check with your physician or physical therapist about which exercises are right for you.

✗ Use a pneumatic pump. These air-driven pumps are used to increase movement of lymphatic fluid. Your arm is placed in a plastic sleeve that fills with air. This added pressure helps move the fluid up your arm. Pumps should be used under the supervision of a therapist.

✗ Maintaining a healthy weight can also help reduce lymphedema.

Lymphedema can be kept under control with a variety of treatments. Tell your physician about any changes in your arm as soon as you notice them. Check with your insurance company to see if your treatment choice is covered.

EXERCISE

There is no question that a mastectomy is a major surgery. Many women experience a great deal of discomfort and stiffness. Fortunately, having a mastectomy rarely causes any permanent limitations in movement, and often, steady exercise can speed up your recovery. However, women who have lost their chest muscles through a radical mastectomy (very uncommon today) might not regain 100 percent of their original strength in the affected arm and shoulder. Still, a regular exercise routine can alleviate some of the tightness in the chest.

Exercise, as was proven in my case, is also very helpful in relieving the symptoms of lymphedema, which is the swelling of the arm following the removal of the lymph nodes in the armpit (axilla).

No exercise program should be contemplated or begun without the expressed consent and guidance of your physician. Your surgeon or physician will recommend specific exercises depending upon your type surgery. You might also contact the "Reach to Recovery" program of the American Cancer Society for exercise information (see the resource section). As soon as your physician gives you the go ahead, a low-key exercise regime should be your next physical goal.

The key is to exercise only to the point where it begins to feel uncomfortable—don't push yourself. Remember, regular exercise will speed your physical recovery, which will enhance your appearance and benefit your emotional recovery.

TAKING CHARGE OF BREAST CANCER

EMOTIONAL RECOVERY

To all of the tips above on prostheses, wigs, makeup, clothing, and exercise, one more must be added. There's a risk factor in your emotional recovery: depression. Depression is anger turned inward. Depression, if it strikes, can cause you to say, "Why bother taking care of myself?" The good news is that there are people who can help you overcome this problem, too. I know that the diagnosis, treatment, and recovery from breast cancer is a stressful period for you and your loved ones. To help you cope through this time, it might be important to seek professional help. Support groups, led by knowledgeable professionals, bring people together to share common experiences. In addition to open discussions where group members share feelings and talk about their progress, most groups also have planned educational sessions. Group facilitators are professionals who have expertise which enables them to provide vital resources and answer your questions. There are even support groups for children and spouses.

"No matter how big or soft or warm your bed is, you still have to get out of it."
Grace Slick

Eventually you may get to a point where coping with breast cancer is no longer an everyday struggle. There are many ways of working through your feelings and moving on with your life. Some activities, like talking to a counselor, help you think through what cancer has meant for you or how it has affected your relationships with others. Other activities, like joining a social club, have nothing to do with cancer, but give you the opportunity to laugh and relax. Think about what kinds of activities might work best for you. You may want to try one or more of these or come up with your own ideas:

Talking
⚐ Continuing to share your feelings with friends and family
⚐ Seeing a counselor, psychologist, or spiritual advisor
⚐ Joining a breast cancer support group
⚐ Joining a breast cancer support chat group on the Internet

Doing
⚐ Taking an art of writing class
⚐ Starting a hobby like yoga or potting
⚐ Studying a foreign language
⚐ Volunteering with an organization

Pampering
⚐ Getting a massage, manicure, or pedicure
⚐ Putting your feet up and reading a good book
⚐ Listening to music

Socializing
⚐ Joining a social group or club (not cancer-related)
⚐ Entertaining friends and family at home
⚐ Asking a friend out to lunch or a movie

Physicians can also prescribe anti-depressants to help you get through what can be a roller coaster ride of emotions ranging from true depression to fear and grief. This is not uncommon. Your emotional makeup is as important as your physical appearance. Remember to take charge of that, too.

Call the American Cancer Society "Reach to Recovery" program, Y-ME, or the Susan G. Komen Breast Cancer Foundation's National Toll-Free Breast Care Helpline at 1.800 I'M AWARE®. See the resource section for contact information. There are understanding, caring people at these organizations who can assist you in finding the help you need. Take advantage of them. You deserve it.

Chapter Eleven
Sexuality and Intimacy

*"Trouble is a part of your life; and if you don't
share it, you don't give the person who loves
you enough chance to love you enough."*
Dinah Shore

When it comes to sexuality, self-image is the name of the game, and both men and women worry about it. For women, it is ingrained in our psyches at an early age through movies, television, books, and magazines that in order to be attractive and desirable to men, we have to have a certain *look.* Flat stomachs, shapely hips, lean legs, and full breasts are the components of a "sexy-looking" woman, so they say. This kind of pressure, we all know, is unhealthy and unfair.

This gender stereotyping becomes particularly difficult for women diagnosed with breast cancer. The ability to retain our sexuality after surgery and hair loss or while ill from the effects of chemotherapy is a constant worry for many women.

Some fear the loss of a breast will make them less than whole, that their altered body will prevent them from ever having a normal life again or keep them from being a complete woman. Because hair loss is only temporary, a woman's fear of it is often dismissed without a lot of psychological evaluation. But I can tell you, through personal experience and through talking with literally thousands of cancer patients, that this fear is a real one. Many women make an emotional connection between their hair and their ability to feel desirable.

Some women are so preoccupied with the thought of losing their sexuality that they will opt to forgo what could be life-saving surgery altogether. My sister Suzy is a prime example. A woman I spoke with in the early days of the Komen Foundation is another. When the Foundation first got off the ground, there were few sources of information or comfort for women diagnosed with breast cancer. In Dallas where I lived, I found myself regularly playing the role of patient advocate, dispensing advice and offering encouragement to many women who had nowhere else to turn.

One night, about two o'clock in the morning, I received a shocking phone call from a woman with breast cancer who was facing a mastectomy. Although her husband had told her repeatedly that the loss of her breast didn't matter to him, she wept as she told me, "I'd rather die than lose my breast." She was convinced if she went ahead with the surgery, her marriage was over. Despite my advice to listen to her husband and get herself to the hospital, she refused to undergo treatment and died a few months later.

On the day my breast cancer was diagnosed, my ultimate concern was to save my life, to get rid of the cancer as thoroughly and as quickly as possible. This was based on my fear of going through the same slow, painful death as Suzy did, and the fact that I was an educated cancer patient. My priorities were pre-established. Every time I had gone in for a biopsy prior to my diagnosis of cancer, I had thought long and hard about what I would do if the tumor was malignant. Still, on that evening before my surgery at M. D. Anderson, sitting in the bed looking at

Norman, I quietly wondered how he would relate to his relatively new wife coming home without a breast. My wonderful friend Sharon McCutchin called me on the telephone and, sensing my concern, said in her long Texas drawl, "Honey, don't worry about it. *That's* not what they really care about, anyway." All I could do was pray she was right.

In the two years that passed between my mastectomy and my reconstruction, I learned a great deal about the true meaning of sexuality. Once again, what works for one woman might not work for another, but I want to share this with you, with the hope of reaching anyone who can possibly benefit from my experience.

At the time, I learned that my ability to be desirable to my husband had little to do with my breasts. I learned that a kind smile, a gentle touch, and a sweet conversation did more for romance than sexy lingerie. From the day we met, Norman and I had always been able to communicate. If we were going to get through this without losing the sparkle, we had to continue to talk openly and honestly about the situation. The truth is that after my surgery and the treatment that followed, quite often I wasn't in the mood for romance. It was up to me to make sure that this was not misinterpreted as lack of love. Norman, being the kind of man he is, understood my feelings. I made it a point to let him know how much I loved him and needed him and to show him that I was trying to get well. Whenever I could help it, and sometimes I couldn't, I tried desperately not to feel sorry for myself and to maintain a cheery disposition. Norman often expressed his pride in my fight to beat the disease. This encouraged me and gave me the incentive to keep trying even on those days when I wanted to give up. His lack of pressure and expectations of me on a sexual level made me try harder to please him.

The fact of the matter is that a mastectomy rarely affects the partner's pleasure or ability to be fulfilled sexually. It is the woman's loss of a sensitive, sexual area that might affect *her* sense of pleasure. There is no reason why, after a few initial adjustments, a couple cannot rekindle a romance that is equally as sensual and full of love as it was before her surgery. Sometimes, when two people acknowledge their own mortality, as a run-in with cancer often forces them to do, their newfound appreciation for life will bring them closer than ever before.

It is vitally important for all women before, during, and after breast cancer to take the time to reevaluate what it means to be a total woman. Is it the size and shape of our breasts and how we look in a bathing suit? Or is it our ability to nurture and protect those we love? For a long time, I have felt that women have an emotional sixth sense; a capability to give open and unconditional love in a deeper, more passionate manner than men will ever have. It is, I think, ingrained in women; a gift we were given naturally; something we have no control over. It is this compassion from which true sexuality is born. Of course, we all want to be thought of as attractive and desirable. But on what is this desirability based? Certainly not on our ability to fill a bra. If we do what we need to do in order to be and feel healthy, eat right, and exercise, we will have the energy it takes to tackle life with spirit. To me, that's what makes a woman sensual. Looking good is usually an added benefit that comes along with doing what it takes to feel good.

"There is no cosmetic for beauty like happiness."
Anonymous

Sometimes, however, eating right and exercising aren't enough to maintain a healthy body. Breast cancer chooses its victims for no apparent rhyme or reason. The healthiest woman in the world can get breast cancer. When this happens she has new choices to make. And sometimes, one of those choices will be to have a mastectomy. If she can get herself in a mind-set to believe that her energy and spirit for living are what make her sexy, she will be much better equipped to handle the emotional and psychological stress involved in losing a breast.

The sexual problems some couples face after a lumpectomy or mastectomy are often the result of preconceived notions on the part of one partner or the other. For example, the man is often afraid to touch the woman after surgery for fear that she might not be up to it or that he might hurt her accidentally in the process. The woman, who has probably already thought herself no longer desirable, might take his lack of overtures as the justification of her feelings. She, then, will be reluctant to initiate a sexual encounter out of fear of further rejection. This is a very common situation and one that can escalate way out of proportion without open and honest communication. As uncomfortable as it is at first, it is in a couple's best interest to resume sexual activity, even on the mildest scale, as soon as possible. If you have tried and just can't seem to muster up the desire for sex after your surgery, or you cannot get a feeling of desire from your partner, you both might want to consider seeing a counselor to open the lines of communication. Or try some of these ideas:

- ⚡ *Take it easy:* Bring some romance back into your life. Plan a relaxing candlelight dinner. Take the time to nurture your sexuality.
- ⚡ *Go slow:* Sometimes just simple affection can be very sexual? Kisses and caresses can provide just as much pleasure.
- ⚡ *Get comfortable:* Sex may be painful if you do not have as much natural lubrication as you are used to. Try using a water-based lubricant like Astroglide® or KY Jelly®.

☒ *Do something different:* Change your sexual routine. Experiment. Try new things. Have some fun.

☒ *Get some advice:* Consider seeking advise from a marriage counselor or joining a support group. You can go with your partner or even by yourself.

But what about the single woman who goes through the mastectomy without a husband or partner? What happens when her surgery is complete, and she feels like getting out there again in the dating circle? When you go through the diagnosis and treatment with a partner, regardless of the difficulties that might ensue, at least you don't have to carry the burden alone. A woman without a partner must keep a private and personal secret inside her while trying to determine the appropriate time to tell a man you are dating that you've had a mastectomy. That's not easy. Obviously, for every couple the situation will be different. Some women like to get it out in the open at the very beginning of a relationship. Others prefer to wait and see if the relationship will progress enough to become intimate at all.

The late Sherri Firnberg, an exuberant young woman actively involved with the Komen Foundation, was, at age twenty-eight, bravely and optimistically beginning treatment for her second recurrence. Sherri was not married, and every time she met a new man, she went through the dilemma of when to tell him. She said, "My first choice is really to keep it a secret. It's not that I have a problem talking about the experience. I don't. But I like to let people see that I'm okay before I start to talk about the cancer. Some people react funny when they hear the word. All of a sudden, they look at you as if you are going to fall apart right in front of them. Unfortunately, though, my secret isn't often a secret for very long. Inevitably, my date and I will run into someone I know, and they'll ask how I'm doing. At that point, I feel sort of obligated to tell. I did meet a man I thought was special. He turned out not to be, but when we first met, we hit it off right away. I immediately felt close to him. I ran over to his house and told him everything. I was relieved when he said it didn't bother him at all. This man was a little older than most of the men I have dated. Maybe it isn't fair to make such a generalization, but so far I have found that older men take the news much better than younger men."

It is important to handle this in a manner that makes you feel comfortable. While constantly talking about it might not be the best way to put the past behind you, your breast cancer and subsequent mastectomy are certainly nothing to be ashamed of. When the situation calls for it, speaking from your heart about your experience can help bring you close to friends in general and perhaps add an element of intimacy and closeness to conversations with potential lovers.

Whether you are happily married, unhappily married, divorced, separated, widowed, or single, one thing is for sure: If you would like to begin or continue a successful sexual relationship, you must first be comfortable with your own self-image. Nobody can give that to you; it must come from within. Remember that dealing with a mastectomy isn't easy for anyone. Your friends, lovers, and children will take their cue from you. If you honestly believe that you are every bit the woman you were before your surgery, so will all who know you and come to know you. And perhaps, if you are lucky, you will find, just as I did, that developing the inner strength to take on cancer as an opponent gives you a sense of femininity you never knew existed. Once you learn that *real* sensuality comes from within the heart and soul, you will also learn that it can never be taken away.

Chapter Twelve
Sharing Your Story
Talking about Breast Cancer

"Loving is not just caring deeply,
it's all about understanding."
Francoise Sagan

As I have mentioned earlier, talking about breast cancer can be difficult. Many people have not been brought up to discuss intimate topics with others comfortably. The intimacy of this disease, coupled with the fear of cancer in general, often creates a communication block within the family, among friends, and at the workplace. The stage of your cancer, combined with your prescribed treatment and how your disease responds to that treatment, will determine the kinds of challenges you are forced to meet along the way.

When and how much to tell your friends, family, and business associates are factors to be considered carefully. As a rule, I feel that honesty is, as always, the best policy. However, you will know better than anyone else in whom you can confide. Having breast cancer is nothing to be embarrassed about. Being surrounded by a close support group will make the ordeal easier and less stressful.

You must be prepared, though, for those who react in an unexpected manner. There are some people who are so afraid and uncomfortable with the word *cancer* that they can't bring themselves to talk about it. Friends, family, and business associates with whom you have always been able to communicate easily might now seem to withdraw just at the time when you need them the most. People who don't understand cancer and how its treatment works are often so afraid of saying the wrong thing, they might say nothing at all. Your first reaction may be to feel hurt. Be patient. Those who love and care about you will also feel like victims of your disease. Their terror and anger over what has happened can manifest itself in unusual ways. Most people will take their lead from you. If you learn to talk honestly, openly, and optimistically about your breast cancer, they will, too. Fair or not, don't be surprised to discover that just when you need to be comforted and nurtured more than at any other time in your life, you are the one doing much of the comforting and nurturing. That, my friends, goes with the territory of being a woman.

For mothers, some of your first thoughts as you were diagnosed, surely included concerns about your children. Should you tell them? What should you tell them? What if they ask you if you are going to die? What will you say? What if you are not around to see them grow? There is nothing abnormal about having these thoughts or any others that might go through your mind. Eric was constantly on my mind from the moment I was diagnosed; every step of the way. The only advice I can give is that whatever you decide to tell your children, try to be as truthful, honest, and open as possible. That is often difficult because our natural instinct as mothers is to protect our children from anything that causes them pain. But remember that children, just like adults, will fill in wherever you leave big gaps. And because children may not know as much as adults, they are more likely to fill the gaps with inaccurate information. Anything that changes their daily routine needs to be explained. Encourage your children to ask questions. Be an anchor for them. You can't maintain the optimistic attitude that is so important to recovery if your children are upset and frightened.

For many families, the trauma of dealing with a life-threatening disease brings them closer than ever before. Bobbye Sloan, the wife of Utah Jazz coach Jerry Sloan, was so protective of her privacy that at first, she kept her diagnosis of breast cancer a secret even from her husband. For most of the six months of her surgery and chemotherapy, she hid from her friends fearing that she would be pitied.

Finally, her son Brian, a physician, got through. "Mom, when are you going to come out of your bedroom?" he asked her. "You have an opportunity to turn something negative into a positive and do some good with what you've been through."

Deep inside, this very private woman knew that her son was right, and her husband felt the same. Bobbye decided to go public. Her first interview was with the Jazz team magazine where she talked about the importance of early detection, mammograms, and monthly breast exams. Once she got her feet wet, there was no stopping Bobbye Sloan's personal crusade against breast cancer.

She did interviews on ESPN, NBC, and *Oprah* to name a few. Jerry was behind her every step of the way—literally. Bobbye and Jerry Sloan became two of the Komen Race for the Cure® Series's biggest supporters. They have run together in Races from Indiana to Utah to the National in Washington. Jerry even quit

> *"When women help women, they help themselves."*
> Wilhelmina Cole Holladay

smoking, and together they remain a pair of very enthusiastic Komen angels.

According to Jerry, "Bobbye said she was going to fight breast cancer like we would fight if we got in the playoffs." To me, Bobbye Sloan and her family will always be All-Stars.

Another friend, Gretchen Poston, handled her situation very differently When Gretchen was diagnosed with breast cancer, she told no one. She went through surgery and chemotherapy all by herself. On the days when the treatment was difficult to endure, she said she wasn't feeling well and stayed at home. She cut her hair short before her chemotherapy began and wore a well-made wig when her hair fell out. Afterward, when Gretchen felt up to it, she did talk about the experience. Her friends were puzzled that she hadn't taken them into her confidence. Gretchen explained that it wasn't a matter of not trusting her friends, it was just that she felt she could get through the ordeal more successfully without worrying that her friends might feel sorry for her. Pity wasn't what Gretchen was looking for.

Another reason my friend Gretchen chose to stay silent was a real concern that some of her clients might feel that she could not carry out her professional responsibilities in her business. Unfortunately, this kind of discrimination does exist. Furthermore, for some women in situations like Gretchen's, pulling the strength and courage to fight from deep inside ultimately gives them a confidence and feeling of self-worth they have never known before.

Because Gretchen was a high-profile Washington, D.C. figure, she did finally go public with her story in 1989. Gretchen lost her battle with breast cancer in January 1992. To honor her memory as the founder of the Komen National Race for the Cure® in Washington, D.C., each year the Race committee gives the Gretchen Poston Award to the Race volunteer who goes above and beyond.

If you have ever attended a Komen Race for the Cure®, you have noticed the sea of pink caps and shirts scattered throughout the crowd. Every time I look at that sight I am reminded of my dear, dear friend, the late Ellen Barnett, who was willing to talk about her breast cancer and who first vocalized the need to celebrate survivorship. Using pink ribbons for breast cancer was her idea, and she conceived of the pink caps as a way to recognize survivors and honor them at Komen Race for the Cure® events. At first, the number of women willing to come forward and wear the caps was small; but as the idea took hold, more and more women survivors began to don the caps and T-shirts and proudly proclaim their survivorship in years, months, and for some, even days. It is inspiring now to see hundreds of pink caps and T-shirts worn by smiling women who are bonded together in a sisterhood of survivorship that only those who have endured breast cancer can know. I thank Ellen Barnett for speaking out and for the gift she gave to the thousands of survivors who run and walk in the Race every year.

As in all matters concerning breast cancer, speaking about it is a personal decision, but I know that I could not have fought the disease as hard as I did without the love and support of my friends. There are certain times and situations in a woman's life when she might be on her own, but there is always someone to talk to. And sometimes, just talking about our fears and frustrations helps us deal with them. You don't have to write a book or appear on television to share your story. But one way you can help other women in the same situation is by becoming a breast cancer advocate. And there are almost as many ways to be an advocate as there are survivors.

You can become an activist—someone who learns all she can about breast cancer and then speaks out publicly. Not everyone likes to get up in front of an audience and tell their story; but by doing so, it helps increase awareness about breast cancer and reach women fighting the disease with a positive message of hope. It also helps get other people involved. For example, raising funds for research, lobbying elected officials, or helping women without in-

surance. You can join a number of different advocacy organizations. See the resource section in this book.

Another type of advocate is a patient advocate. Some
hospitals have a volunteer program in which women who
have had breast cancer visit women newly diagnosed
with the disease. If your hospital or community does not
have such a program, consider starting one.

You can also be an advocate by writing an article for
your local newspaper. It can help you keep a positive,
determined attitude, and your story might inspire someone else to persevere.

The women I know who have not only been successful in fighting breast cancer but have been an inspiration
to other cancer patients, have known when to discuss
their problems and when to keep silent. There is a time
and place for both. Remember, there is a difference
between developing the ability to talk openly and honestly about the disease and unloading your anger, fear,
and confusion onto anyone who happens to cross your
path. Advocacy and anger have their place in any breast
cancer patient's life. I found it always helps to try to
strike a balance between fighting the disease publicly and
saving enough strength for the very personal fight.
Today, breast cancer is much more widely discussed than
in the past, thanks to the Komen Foundation and organizations like it. We've taken breast cancer out of the shadows and into the streets.

Chapter Thirteen
If Cancer Recurs

"You may have to fight a battle more than once to win it."
Margaret Thatcher

RECOMMENDATIONS FOR FOLLOW-UP CARE

The American Society of Clinical Oncology has established the following guidelines for follow-up of breast cancer treatment:

- Have a physical examination performed by a doctor every three to six months during the first three years after treatment; every six to twelve months for the next two years; and once a year after that
- Perform a breast self-exam every month
- Have a mammogram every year
- Understand the symptoms of cancer recurrence
- Have a Pap smear and gynecological examination every year

When breast cancer is first diagnosed, fear, anger, confusion, and desperation seem to take over in the beginning as the realization of our own mortality sinks in. As a woman learns more about her options and understands all that can be done to combat the disease, some of those emotions are replaced by hope and an overwhelming feeling of strength and determination. Ideally, you will

TAKING CHARGE OF BREAST CANCER

get through the ordeal and will gain a better appreciation for life as you live each new day to the fullest.

It doesn't always happen that way. After bravely enduring one or more types of treatment, even the most noble of fighters can be faced with the devastating news that her cancer has recurred. A recurrent cancer is a tumor growth in the area of the original cancer site, either in the remaining breast tissue, the skin, the chest wall, or nearby lymph nodes. It might also be a form of metastasis, cancer that has spread through the blood and/or lymph system to other parts of the body such as the bones, liver, lungs, or brain. It is possible that some of the original cancer cells were not destroyed by the first round of treatment. They might have lain dormant for several months or even years before beginning a regrowth.

SOME SYMPTOMS OF CANCER RECURRENCE

- ✗ These include any changes in the remaining breast(s) and chest area, unusual pain, loss of appetite or weight, unusual vaginal bleeding, or blurred vision.
- ✗ Dizziness, coughing that does not go away, hoarseness, shortness of breath, headaches, backaches, or digestive problems that are unusual or that do not go away.
- ✗ Any unusual symptoms should be reported to the doctor, who will examine you and determine the nature of the symptoms.

Recommendations for Follow-Up Care

Having a breast cancer recurrence is not necessarily a death sentence. Many women go on to live full, healthy, and active lives after one or more cancer recurrences. Still, the emotional energy required to gear up again for more treatment after believing that you have beaten the disease can be staggering. A feeling of bitter disappointment combined with rage and despair can be crippling if you allow it to be. This is the time when you will need every bit of courage and positive energy you can muster. "Know, above all else, that this is not your fault," insists Dr. Jimmie Holland of Memorial Sloan-Kettering in New York. "Release the guilt. A cancer recurrence is not a personal failure, it is a disease."

The treatment options for breast cancer recurrence are the same as for initial breast cancer. If the initial surgery was less extensive, more surgery might be required. Chemotherapy, radiation therapy, and/or hormone therapy might also be suggested, although the dosages might vary according to your specific need.

Should you be diagnosed with recurrent or metastatic disease, your medical team of experts as well as your emotional support system will need to come up with a new strategy and a new plan of action. Try to find strength in the fact that by now you are a much more knowledgeable and educated cancer patient. Some of the mystery and uncertainty about what to expect from the treatment will be diminished. Knowing what to expect will enable you to better organize your next round of treatment around the rest of your life.

And it is important to go on being as active as possible. Don't give up or give in to this disease. This time you might beat it—once and for all. Remember, others have done it successfully before you. I know many people who have lived sometimes years beyond a medical diagnosis through sheer will and faith. Just stay focused on what you have learned to do to help yourself and stay positive.

> *"Never give in. Never, never, never, never."*
> **Winston Churchill**

If you do not personally know a patient who has survived recurrent or metastatic breast cancer, contact the

Susan G. Komen Breast Cancer Foundation, the American Cancer Society, or Y-ME; these organizations will be able to put you in touch with someone in your area who can give you, firsthand, the hope and courage you need to go on.

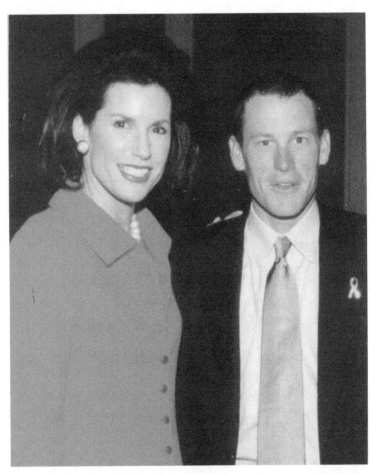

Olympic athlete, two-time Tour de France winner, and testicular cancer survivor Lance Armstrong joins Nancy Brinker as a presenter at the Komen Foundation National Awards Luncheon. Armstrong's triumph over cancer and his winning attitude serve as an inspiration to everyone.

Chapter Fourteen
Breast Cancer and Priority Populations

"It's always something."
Gilda Radner

ETHNIC POPULATIONS

Anyone can develop breast cancer. Even men. But if you are a woman, you already have the leading risk factor for getting breast cancer just by being a woman. And as you grow older, you have the number two risk factor—increasing age. Breast cancer is one of the most common cancers among women in the U.S. It is the most frequently diagnosed cancer among nearly every female racial and ethnic group, including African-American, Alaskan Native, American Indian, Chinese, Filipino, Hawaiian/Pacific Islander, Hispanic, Japanese, and Korean women.

For white women over the age of forty, their ethnicity puts them in the highest risk groups for getting breast cancer. But for some populations, particularly older women of color, their ethnicity may not put them at higher risk of *getting* breast cancer, but their chances of having their cancer detected early and getting the treatment they need are lower because of psychosocial barriers unique to their groups. Medically-underserved women, for example, may not have access to regular healthcare, breast health information, or screening facilities.

This lack of access translates into higher mortality rates. African-American women are less likely than Caucasian women to survive for five years after being diagnosed with breast cancer and more likely to die from breast cancer. In addition, we are seeing larger numbers of Hispanic women with breast cancer due to their population growth rate. And when Asian women migrate to the U.S., their risk of developing breast cancer increases up to six-fold. Asian immigrant women living in the U.S. for as little as a decade had an 80 percent higher risk of breast cancer than new immigrants. Clearly, we have a big education job ahead of us if we are going to change the odds for priority populations.

> *"America is not a melting pot but a Mosaic."*
> Pat Derian

YOUNG WOMEN AND BREAST CANCER

For other populations, such as men and younger women, it may be a misguided notion that they simply can't get breast cancer because of their age or sex. Why do "young" women get breast cancer? When it comes to breast cancer, "young" usually means anyone younger than forty years old. Breast cancer is less common among women in this age group. In 1999, only 5 percent of all breast cancer cases occurred in women under age forty. However, women who are diagnosed at a younger age are likely to have a mutated BRCA1 or BRCA2 gene. These genes are important in the development of breast cancer, and women who carry defects on either of these genes are at a greater risk of developing breast and ovarian cancer. In addition, having a mother, daughter, or sister who has or had breast cancer also increases a young woman's risk of developing breast cancer. If a woman has both a family history and carries the defective BRCA1 or BRCA2 gene, she may have a 50 to 85 percent chance of developing breast cancer in her lifetime. So while the risk of breast cancer is generally much lower for younger women, there is still a high risk for some.

If you are concerned with your genetic risk, ask your physician to refer you to a genetic counselor or a breast cancer specialist who will discuss in detail what your own risk may be and can discuss prevention options. Diagnosing breast cancer in younger women can be more difficult because their breast tissue is often denser than older women's. By the time a lump can be felt in a younger woman, it is sometimes large enough and advanced enough to lower her chances of survival. That was certainly what happened to Suzy.

In addition, the cancer may be more aggressive and less responsive to hormone therapies. Delay of diagnosis in younger women is a special problem because it is much less common for a younger woman to get the disease. As a result, younger women are often told that a lump is just a cyst and to wait and watch it. Tell your physician if you notice a change in either of your breasts, and think about getting a second opinion if you are not satisfied with his or her advice.

BREAST CANCER IN MEN

Breast cancer in men is rare, but it does happen. After all, men have breast tissue also. In the U.S., fewer than 1 in 100,000 men are diagnosed with breast cancer each year. Although that sounds like a small number, roughly 1,300 men are diagnosed and about 400 die of the disease in the United States every year. Several factors increase a man's risk of getting breast cancer. Some of these have been strongly linked with breast cancer in men, others have a weaker link to breast cancer, and the specific roles of others are still under research. These factors include:

❧ Getting older
❧ Having family members (male or female) with breast cancer, especially with a BRCA2 mutation.
❧ Having your chest area exposed to radiation treatment
❧ Taking estrogen for a sex change
❧ Having higher levels of female hormones called estrogen (common with liver diseases such as cirrhosis).
❧ Having a genetic condition such as Klinefelter's syndrome.

WOMEN WHO PARTNER WITH WOMEN AND LESBIANS

Women who partner with women and lesbians do have a greater risk of breast cancer than other women, but not because of their sexual orientation or their genetic make-up. Again, psychosocial barriers come into play. First, most of these women don't have children, which puts them at higher risk for getting the disease. Second, because they don't have children, a higher number may not seek the regular gynecological care that reproductive concerns often generate in heterosexual women.

For many women, reproductive health issues are their main link to the health care system. Even when they see a physician about reproductive health, women often discuss other health issues, including having a clinical breast exam or mammogram. Because lesbians may have fewer opportunities to have similar discussions and screening, breast cancer may not be detected as early as possible among lesbians.

If you are a lesbian, breast health is just as important for you as any other woman. Find a physician who is sensitive to your health issues and make clinical breast exams and mammograms part of your routine.

The Komen Foundation continues to research, develop, and implement new outreach opportunities among priority populations and to look for further ways to increase the effectiveness of our current programs for priority populations. In addition, our local Komen Affiliates fund non-duplicative community-based breast health education and breast cancer screening and treatment projects for the medically underserved that do a wonderful job at reaching women at special risk.

If you are a member of a priority population, take advantage of these and other programs designed to meet your needs. They can help you take control of your life and care.

CONCLUSION

For me, this book is part of a promise kept. For you, I hope it has been the friend that I meant it to be. I wrote it to give you comfort in the down times; to give you hope and courage and crucial information. No doubt, not every question or concern that you might have has been answered, but now you have the tools to know where to go for help and what to ask.

This is a book about living, not dying; about never giving up or giving in because Suzy would have wanted it that way. So, make a promise to yourself to take charge of your care and live!

Breast Health Glossary

There are some terms you will see over and over again within this book and hear often in your doctor's office. I have tried to explain each term as it came up in the text, but I know from experience that "cancer talk" can sound like a foreign language at first. And foreign languages are easy to forget. The Susan G. Komen Breast Cancer Foundation has put together a quick reference list of common terms to refresh your memory at a glance. The definitions are short and uncomplicated, meant only to give you a fast, easy idea of what a word means. For more detailed information, use the index to find the term within the text, or ask your physician.

Adjuvant Therapy: cancer treatment such as chemotherapy or hormone therapy, used in addition to the primary form of treatment, which is generally surgery.

Alopecia: hair loss. Often occurs as a result of chemotherapy.

Alternative Therapy: any non-traditional cancer treatment used instead of a traditional medical cancer treatment.

Anesthesia: entire or partial loss of feeling or sensation produced by drugs or gases (temporary).

Antiemetic: a medicine used to prevent or relieve nausea and vomiting.

Areola: darkly shaded area that encircles the nipple.

Aspiration: withdrawal of fluid from a cyst with a hypodermic needle.

Atypical Hyperplasia: increased growth of abnormal cells.

Axilla: the underarm area.

Axillary Lymph Nodes: glands in the underarm that filter the lymph fluid.

Benign: biopsy result indicating that cancer is not present in the cells of a breast mass.

Biopsy: test used to remove cellular tissue so that it can be examined under a microscope to look for cancerous cells.

Bone (skeletal) Survey: X rays of the entire skeleton.

Bone Scan: a picture of all the bones in the body taken two hours after injection of a radioactive tracer.

BRCA1 & BRCA2: human genes which, when present in a mutated form, increase a woman's risk of developing breast and ovarian cancer.

Breast Cancer: an uncontrolled growth of abnormal breast cells.

Breast Conserving Surgery (lumpectomy): surgery in which minimal breast tissue is removed—usually only the tumor and a small surrounding area of normal tissue.

Breast Implant: an envelope containing silicone or saline (or both) surgically inserted to restore breast form.

Breast Self-Examination (BSE): screening that involves examining one's own breast for lumps and changes.

Cancer: diseases involving abnormal uncontrolled cell growth that can spread throughout the body.

CAT Scan: a cross-sectional view of the entire body through X ray that might show cancer or metastases earlier and more accurately than other imaging methods.

Chemotherapy: the use of drugs to treat cancer by destroying or slowing the growth of cancer cells.

Clinical Breast Examination (CBE): breast exam performed by a trained medical professional that includes visual examination and palpation (feeling) of the entire breast to check for any physical changes or lumps in the breast.

Clinical Trials: research studies conducted with actual patients to examine the safety and effectiveness of new drugs or treatments.

Complementary Therapy: any non-traditional cancer treatment that is used together with traditional medical cancer treatment.

Core Needle Biopsy: removal of a cylinder of tissue with a thicker, hollow needle from a growth or mass for microscopic diagnosis. Sometimes referred to as stereotactic biopsy.

Cyst: a fluid-filled sac or cavity, usually harmless, which can be removed by aspiration. See *aspiration*.

Cytotoxic: cell-killing.

Diagnostic Tests: tests used to determine the nature of breast changes.

Duct Ectasia: see *mammary duct ectasia*.

Ductal Papilloma: noncancerous breast tumor, arising in the breast duct, usually cannot be felt. Commonly found in women forty-five to fifty. Generally causes either a bloody or clear nipple discharge.

Ducts: channels that transport milk from the lobules to the nipple.

Endocrine Manipulation: treating breast cancer by depriving breast cancer cells of the hormone they need to live.

Estrogen: a female reproductive hormone.

Estrogen Receptor Assay (ERA): a laboratory test performed on a malignant breast tumor to determine if the tumor's growth is responsive to estrogen.

Excisional Biopsy: removal of an entire growth for diagnosis.

Fat Narcosis: hard lumps that are formed by damaged fatty tissue.

Fat Necrosis: destruction of fat cells due to trauma or injury that can cause a noncancerous lump.

Fibroadenomas: round, rubbery, benign tumors.

Fibrocystic Breast Changes: lumpiness in the breast and tenderness or pain at certain times of the month.

Fibrocystic Breast Condition: a noncancerous breast condition sometimes resulting in painful cysts or lumpy breasts. It can be accompanied by discomfort or pain that fluctuates with menstrual cycle.

Fine Needle Aspiration Biopsy: removal of cells or fluid with a small diameter needle, from a growth or mass for microscopic diagnosis.

Frozen Section: a technique in which a part of the biopsy tissue is frozen immediately and a thin slice is then mounted on a microscope slide, enabling a pathologist to analyze it in just a few minutes for a diagnosis.

Halsted (Radical) Mastectomy: see *Mastectomy*.

Hormone Receptor Assay: a diagnostic test to determine whether a breast cancer's growth is influenced by hormones and can be treated with hormone therapy.

Hormone Therapy: treatment that blocks your body's natural hormones from stimulating the growth of any remaining cancer cells.

Hormones: chemicals produced by various glands in the body.

Hysterectomy: surgical removal of the uterus.

Immunotherapy: treatment of cancer by stimulating the body's immune defense system.

In Situ: abnormal cell growth that stays in the place of origin; opposite of invasive.

Incisional Biopsy: surgical removal of a portion of a growth or mass for microscopic diagnosis.

Infiltrating Duct Cell Cancer: a cancer that begins in the mammary ducts and spreads to surrounding breast tissue. (Also called infiltrating ductal carcinoma.)

Intravenous (IV): entering the body by way of a vein.

Invasive Cancer: the spread of cancer from the location where it started into surrounding tissue.

Inverted Nipple: the turning inward of the nipple. Usually a condition present from early in life, but if it occurs where it has not previously existed, it can be a sign of breast cancer.

Latissimus Dorsi Flap Reconstruction: the latissimus dorsi, a large, flat muscle on the patient's back, along with the overlying skin, is used to reconstruct a breast mound at the mastectomy site. The patient might require an expander or implant if there is not enough tissue to achieve an appropriate volume.

Lobules: milk-producing glands in the breasts.

Lump: any kind of mass in the breast (or elsewhere in the body).

Lumpectomy: a surgical procedure in which only the cancerous tumor and a ring of surrounding normal breast tissue are removed, leaving the remaining normal breast tissue intact. Usually some of the underarm lymph nodes are removed with another incision. This procedure is followed by radiation.

Lumpy Breasts: see *fibrocystic breast condition*.

Lymph Nodes: glands, found throughout the body, that filter the lymph fluid, removing wastes and fluids from the body tissues and along with white blood cells help the body fight infection. Those found in the underarm (axilla) are most likely to be invaded by breast cancer cells and therefore some are removed during breast cancer surgery.

Lymphedema: swelling in the arm caused by excess fluid that might occur after lymph nodes and vessels have been removed during surgery or following radiation therapy.

Magnetic Resonance Imaging (MRI): a magnet scan; a form of X ray using magnets instead of radiation. MRI gives a more clearly defined picture of fatty tissue than X ray.

Malignant: biopsy result indicating that cancer is present in a breast mass.

Mammary Duct Ectasia: a noncancerous breast condition resulting from the inflammation and enlargement of the ducts behind the nipple. Generally women are asymptomatic (no symptoms); however, mammographic calcifications might indicate its presence. No treatment is necessary if the woman is not experiencing any symptoms (burning, pain, or itching of the nipple area).

Mammary Glands: the breast glands that produce and carry milk, by way of the mammary ducts, to the nipples during pregnancy and breast-feeding.

Mammography/Mammogram: an X-ray picture of the breast for screening and diagnosis of breast cancer.

    ✗ A *baseline mammogram* is an initial screening mammogram to establish a basis for comparison to subsequent mammograms

    ✗ A *diagnostic mammogram* is an X ray taken to further evaluate an already palpable lump or some other abnormality or an abnormality found on a screening mammogram

    ✗ A *screening mammogram* is an X ray taken in an asymptomatic (no symptoms) woman to detect any abnormality that might indicate early signs of breast cancer

Mastectomy: surgery in which the entire breast is removed, along with some or all axillary lymph nodes.

Medical Oncologist: a physician who specializes in the treatment of cancer using chemotherapy or hormone therapy.

Menopause: the time in a woman's life when the menstrual cycle ends, and the ovaries produce lower levels of hormones. Usually occurs between the ages of 45 and 55, but may occur earlier.

Metastasis: the spread of cancer cells from the location where it started to other parts of the body.

Microsurgery: the suturing and reattachment of blood vessels under the magnification of the operating microscope; technique often used in breast reconstruction.

Modified Radical Mastectomy: the most common type of mastectomy performed today. The breast, breast skin, nipple, areola, and underarm lymph nodes are removed, while the chest muscles are saved

Neoadjuvant therapy: chemotherapy or radiation therapy given before surgery to reduce the size of a tumor.

Nipple Discharge: secretions or fluid coming from the nipple.

Oncogenes: an abnormally functioning gene that can cause unregulated cell growth that leads to the formation of a tumor.

Oncologist: a doctor who specializes in treating cancer.

One-Step Procedure: a procedure in which a surgical biopsy is performed under general anesthesia and, if cancer is found, a mastectomy or lumpectomy is done immediately as part of the same operation. It should be noted that this is no longer the standard procedure unless the patient is informed and consents in advance to a one-step procedure.

Oophorectomy: surgical removal of the ovaries.

Palliative Therapy: a treatment that might relieve symptoms without curing the disease.

Partial Mastectomy: see *segmental mastectomy*.

Pathologist: a physician with special training in diagnosing diseases from samples of tissues.

Palpation: (feeling) examining with the hands to check for changes or abnormalities.

Permanent Section: a technique in which thin slices of biopsy tissue are mounted on a slide to be examined under a microscope by a pathologist in order to establish a diagnosis. Usually takes three working days to receive the final pathology report.

Progesterone Receptor Assay (PRA): a test that must be done on cancerous tissue to see if a breast cancer is hormone-dependent and can be treated by hormone therapy. Used as a check on the results of the estrogen receptor assay.

Prognosis: the likelihood that a woman will recover from breast cancer.

Proliferative Rate: a test done on cancerous tissue to determine the growth rate of malignant cells. Indicates aggressiveness of tumor.

Prophylactic Mastectomy: a procedure that removes one or both breasts, sometimes recommended for patients at very high risk for developing cancer in one or both breasts. Refer to *mastectomy*.

Prosthesis, Breast: an external breast form that can be worn underneath clothing after a mastectomy.

Radiation Oncologist: a physician specifically trained in the use of high-energy X rays to treat cancer.

Radiation Therapy (radiotherapy): treatment using high-energy X rays to destroy cancer cells.

Radical Mastectomy (Halsted Radical): the surgical removal of the breast, breast skin, nipple, areola, chest muscles, and underarm lymph nodes. Rarely done today.

Radiologist: a physician who specializes in diagnosis of diseases by the use of X rays.

Receptor: a specific location in a cancer cell that attracts hormones to attach to it in order to promote growth.

Reconstructive Surgery: a procedure using plastic surgery to recreate a breast.

Recurrence: a return of breast cancer in your body at either the same site (local), near the site (regional), or in other areas of the body (metastatic or distant).

Risk Factors: factors that affect a woman's chances of getting breast cancer.

Screening: a test or procedure used to detect cancer in a person who does not have symptoms.

Segmental Mastectomy (Partial Mastectomy): a surgical procedure in which only a portion of the breast is removed, including the cancer and a surrounding margin of healthy breast tissue. See also *lumpectomy*.

Stages of Cancer: a numbering system (from 0 to 4) that tells doctors how advanced a specific breast cancer may be in order to determine appropriate treatment options.

Subcutaneous Mastectomy: removes the breast tissue but leaves the outer skin, areola, and nipple intact. (Not performed very often.)

Tamoxifen: a drug used to block estrogen from stimulating cancer cells to grow.

Transverse Rectus Abdominus Myocutaneous Flap (TRAM): To create a breast mound, the surgeon transfers one of the two abdominal muscles, technically called Transverse Rectus Abdominus Myocutaneous, from the stomach to the chest. This procedure is commonly called a TRAM. This flap of muscle, skin, and fat is shaped into the contour of the opposite breast. If there is enough abdominal tissue available, no implant is needed. This procedure also tightens the abdominal muscles, giving rise to the term "tummy tuck" procedure. The patient will have a scar across the lower abdomen in addition to the mastectomy scar on her chest. Because there are, in effect, two surgeries being performed, recovery might be prolonged.

Tumor: an uncontrolled growth of cells that are either benign or malignant.

Two-Step Procedure: when surgical biopsy and further surgical treatment are performed at two separate times. Compare to *one-step procedure*.

Ultrasonography/Ultrasound: a noninvasive procedure (a procedure that does not require cutting into the skin) using a sound wave imaging technique to examine the breast. Ultrasound might be helpful in distinguishing between solid masses and cysts. Unlike mammography, ultrasound cannot detect micro calcifications that might be present in the breast.

X rays: electromagnetic radiation, which can, at low levels, produce images that can diagnose cancer and, at high levels, destroy cancer cells.

Resource Section

The following list of breast health and breast cancer organizations is provided by the Susan G. Komen Breast Cancer Foundation solely as a suggested resource. However, please note that this is not a complete listing of breast health and breast cancer organizations and that this information is not meant to be used for self-diagnosis or to replace the services of a medical professional. Further, the Komen Foundation does not recommend, endorse, or make any warranties or representations regarding the accuracy, quality, or appropriateness of any of the materials, products, or information provided by the organizations referred to in this list.

The Susan G. Komen Breast Cancer Foundation
5005 LBJ Freeway Suite 250
Dallas, Texas 75244
1.800 I'M AWARE® (1-800-462-9273)
Se habla español. TDD available.
www.breastcancerinfo.com

The Susan G. Komen Breast Cancer Foundation fights to eradicate breast cancer by advancing research, education, screening, and treatment. The Komen Foundation provides a Toll-Free Breast Care Helpline that is answered by trained, caring volunteers whose lives have been personally touched by breast cancer.

American Cancer Society (ACS)
1599 Clifton Road, NE
Atlanta, Georgia 30329
1-800-ACS-2345
www.cancer.org

Provides information and resources; the Reach to Recovery Program trains breast cancer survivors who visit newly diagnosed post-surgical patients.

AMC Cancer Research Center
1600 Pierce St.
Denver, CO 80214
1-800-525-3777
www.amc.org

The AMC Cancer Research Center provides information on symptoms, diagnosis, treatment, psychosocial issues, support groups and other valuable resources, such as financial aid and transportation services.

American College of Radiology
Mammography Accreditation Program
1891 Preston White Drive
Reston, Virginia 22091
1-800-227-6440
www.acr.org

Provides lists of facilities with accredited mammography units.

American Medical Association (AMA)
515 North State Street
Chicago, Illinois 60610
312-464-5000
www.ama-assn.org

The American Medical Association serves to promote the art and science of medicine and the betterment of public health.

American Society of Clinical Oncology (ASCO)
1900 Duke Street
Suite 200
Alexandria, VA 22314
703-299-0150
www.asco.org

Resource for oncology professionals and cancer patients.

American Society of Plastic and Reconstructive Surgeons
444 East Algonquin Road
Arlington Heights, Illinois 60005
1-888-475-2784
www.plasticsurgery.org

An information and referral service for individuals seeking the services of a board-certified plastic surgeon, including those who perform breast reconstruction procedures.

Cancer Care
Cancer Care, Inc. National Office
275 7th Ave
New York, NY 10001

1-800-813-HOPE
www.cancercare.org

Offers free counseling and emotional support, information about cancer and treatments, financial assistance, educational seminars, and referral to other support groups.

Cancer Information and Counseling Line
1600 Pierce St.
Denver, CO 80214
1-800-525-3777
www.cicl.amc.org

Established in 1981 by AMC Cancer Research Center, the CICL is a national toll-free telephone information line designed to help people with cancer and their families.

Food and Drug Administration's Breast Implant Information Line
FDA Office of Device Evaluation
Division of General Restorative and Neurological Devices
9200 Corporate Blvd.
HF2-410
Rockville, MD 20850
1-888-INFO FDA
www.fda.gov/cdrh/breastimplants/indexbip.html

Provides free comprehensive information packages about breast implants.

"Look Good-Feel Better"
American Cancer Society
1599 Clifton Road, NE
Atlanta, GA 30329
1-800-395-LOOK (1-800-395-5665)
www.cancer.org

Program designed to help women recovering from cancer deal with changes in their appearance resulting from cancer treatment. Print and video material available.

The Mautner Project for Lesbians with Cancer
HO 2010 1707 L Street NW, Suite 500
Washington, DC 20036
202-332-5536
www.mautnerproject.org

Provides education, support and other services to lesbians with cancer and their partners.

National Alliance of Breast Cancer Organizations (NABCO)
9 East 37th Street lOth Floor
New York, NY 10016
1-888-80-NABCO
www.nabco.org

NABCO provides lists of national breast cancer support groups.

National Breast Cancer Coalition
1707 L Street, NW
Suite 1060
Washington D.C. 20036
1-800-622-2838
www.natlbcc.org

A grassroots organization with a mission to eradicate breast cancer through action and advocacy.

National Cancer Institute (NCI)/Cancer Information Service
NCI Public Inquiries Office
Building, #31, Room 2B10
9000 Rockville Pike
Bethesda, MD 20892
1-800-4-CANCER (1-800-422-6237)
www.cancernet.nci.nih.gov

NCI's Cancer Information Service provides information and resources for patients, the public and health care providers.

National Center for Complementary and Alternative Medicine at the National Institutes of Health
P.O. Box 8218
Silver Spring, Maryland 20907-8218
1-888-644-6226
www.nccam.nih.gov

Provides information on complementary and alternative health care.

National Coalition for Cancer Survivorship (NCCS)
1010 Wayne Avenue
Suite 770
Silver Spring, Maryland 20910

1-877-622-7937
www.cansearch.org

NCCS is a network of independent organizations and individuals working in the areas of cancer support and survivorship. The primary goal of the coalition is to generate a nationwide awareness of cancer survivorship.

The National Hospice and Palliative Care Organization
1700 Diagonal Road, Suite 300
Alexandria, VA 22314
703-837-1500
www.nhpco.org

A nonprofit organization and the nation's only advocate for terminally ill patients and their families. Member programs and services include advocacy, educational events and symposia, technical assistance, public relations support, legislative bulletins, and several publications.

National Insurance Consumer Helpline
Insurance Information Institute
Publication Service
110 Williams Street
New York, NY 10038
1-800-942-4242
www.iii.org

Trained personnel and licensed agents are available to assist consumers in three important areas. They answer a wide range of questions about various insurance matters, are able to refer consumer complaints to appropriate sources, and send consumer brochures upon request.

National Lymphedema Network
Latham Square
1611 Telegraph Avenue
Suite 1111
Oakland, CA 94612-2138
1-800-541-3259
www.lymphnet.org

A nonprofit organization that disseminates information on the prevention and management of primary and secondary lymphedema to the general public and healthcare professionals, and supports research into the causes, prevention, and management of lymphedema.

National Society of Genetic Counselors, Inc.
www.nsgc.org

Patient Advocate Foundation
753 Thimble Shoals Blvd., Suite B
Newport News, VA 23606
1-800-532-5274
www.patientadvocate.org

A national nonprofit organization that serves as an active liaison between the patient and their insurer, employer and/or creditors.

Physicians Data Query (PDQ)-A division of National Cancer Institute (NCI)/
Cancer Information Service
Bldg. # 31, Room 2B10
9000 Rockville Pike
Bethesda, MD 20892
1-800-4-CANCER (1-800-422-6237)
www.nci.nih.gov

A computer database of the NCI that provides cancer information statements, descriptions of research studies, listings of organizations involved in cancer care, and summaries of clinical trials.

Y-ME National Breast Cancer Organization
212 W. Van Buren, Suite 500
Chicago, Illinois 60607
1-800-221-2141 or 1 800-986-9505 (Spanish)
www.y-me.org

The mission of Y-ME National Breast Cancer Organization is to decrease the impact of breast cancer, create and increase breast cancer awareness, and to ensure, through information, empowerment, and peer support, that no one faces breast cancer alone.

YWCA Encore Plus Program
Empire State Bldg., Suite 301
350 Fifth Avenue
New York, NY 10118
212-273-7800
www.ywca.org

Encore Plus is a breast and cervical cancer outreach and screening program for women over 50.

Partners in the Promise

Twenty years ago, I promised my sister Suzy that I would do everything I could to put an end to breast cancer. I planted the seed of that promise by founding the Susan G. Komen Breast Cancer Foundation in my sister's memory in 1982. Now, twenty years later, the Komen Foundation is a leading catalyst in the fight against breast cancer, with roots stretching around the globe. Our branches are far reaching in large part because of the many generous corporate partners we have worked with along the way. Through the warmth of their care, our corporate partners have nurtured the progress of the promise. They have made the cause their own and have become partners in the truest sense of the word. They are the lifeblood of the Komen family tree and together, we will continue to work until a cure is found and the promise fulfilled.

The Komen Foundation is extremely proud to partner with these generous corporations and organizations:

*American Airlines
*American Express
American Golf Association
American Taekwondo Association
Applause, Inc.
Aventis
*BMW of North America
Boise Cascade
Brinker International
Bristol-Myers Squibb
Danskin
Day-Timers
Deluxe Financial Services
Ethicon-Endo Surgery
Ford Credit
*Ford Division
GE Medical
Gillette
Golden Valley Foods
Goldsmith Seeds
Halcyon Enamels
*Hallmark
Harrah's
Home Sewing Association
Jane Blaylock and Company
Jazzercise
JCPenney
*Johnson & Johnson
*Kellogg's
KitchenAid
Ladies Professional Golf Association
*Lee Jeans
Mohawk Carpets
National Football League

Neiman Marcus
New Balance Athletic Shoe
*Occidental Chemical
Parade of Shoes
Pier 1 Imports
Proflowers.com
Republic of Tea
Saks Fifth Avenue
Samsung
Sprint
Talbot's
TexStyle Home Fashions
The Bombay Company
The Carlisle Collection
*The Wrenfield Group/Rally for a Cure
*Titleist & Footjoy Worldwide
Tropicana
Turtle Creek Chorale
Uncle Ben's
U.S. Women's Synchronized Swim Team
Val Skinner – Life Event
Wacoal
Women's Chorus of Dallas
Women's International Bowling Congress
*Women's Motorcyclist Foundation
Wyndham International
*Yoplait
Zeneca Pharmaceuticals Group
*Zeta Tau Alpha Fraternity

Asterisk indicates a member of the Susan G. Komen Breast Cancer Foundation's Million Dollar Council.

Index